DEAFNESS IN THE FAMILY

Advisory Editor: Daniel Ling, Ph.D.

Deafness in the Family

DAVID LUTERMAN, D.Ed.

Professor, Communication Disorders
Emerson College
Boston, Massachusetts

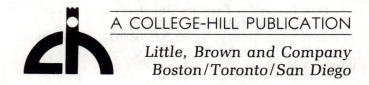

A COLLEGE-HILL PUBLICATION

Little, Brown and Company
Boston/Toronto/San Diego

College-Hill Press
A Division of
Little, Brown and Company (Inc.)
34 Beacon Street
Boston, Massachusetts 02108

Library of Congress Cataloging in Publication Data
Main entry under title:

  Luterman, David.
    Deafness in the family.

    Includes bibliographies and index.
    1. Children, Deaf—Family relationships—Case studies.
  I. Title. [DNLM: 1. Deafness—in infancy & childhood.
  2. Family. WV 271 L973d]
  HV2392.2.L87   1987   362.4'2'088054   86–29882

ISBN 0–316–53754–3

Printed in the United States of America.

This book is dedicated to my wife Carolyn and our four children, Alison, Daniel, Emily, and James, my own nuclear family, which is dissolving and re-forming in interesting ways.

This book is dedicated to my wife Carole and our four children, Joseph, Damien, Reilly, and Karen... we hope... and continue... with their talents and to continue in the coming years.

CONTENTS

FOREWORD

This book is about families and how they may be affected by childhood hearing impairment. In writing this text, David Luterman has drawn on his extensive experience in counseling to analyse the reactions to deafness in three families he came to know intimately. He has complemented this experience with his exceptional talents as a scholar and an astute observer. The outcome is a text that will help readers, whatever their backgrounds, to understand the dynamics of change that occur in families when children are discovered to have—and must learn to live with—serious auditory deficits.

No single text can deal adequately with every type of family. This book is about the sorts of families that any reader might meet or know. It does not set out to deal with families in which the parents are deaf. Such a book has yet to be written.

Families are complex units. Nevertheless, Dr. Luterman has found a way to write about families and the impact upon them in a simple manner. Much as he brings child, siblings, parents, and grandparents into focus in different chapters of the book, so does he weave their interactions into each chapter. This treatment allows the reader to perceive and understand the nature and abundance of adjustments that must be made by a family in order to preserve its balance and provide its members with opportunities to grow.

The hearing-impaired children in the families depicted in this book are all now young adults. Much of the material from the interviews recorded is therefore retrospective. Since clarity of vision is often best yielded by hindsight, this perspective is advantageous for those readers who are in the earlier stages of coping with deafness in the family.

This is a book that will entertain as well as teach the reader. It does not set out to provide hope or encouragement to families faced with deafness in a child, but hope and encouragement emerge as by-products in this account of how human beings function in the face of adversity.

Daniel Ling, Ph.D.
Dean, Faculty of Applied Health Sciences
University of Western Ontario
London, Ontario

Families and family have always been very important to me. I am not sure what in my upbringing shaped me into having that strong a value. I can recall feeling as a child that the worst villain in all of literature was Hansel's and Gretel's father because he allowed his children to be abandoned. To this day I cannot abide that story.

This has also been a very emotional time for me as my fourth and last child is preparing to leave home, and my own parents are aging. I can hear the clang of the changing of the guard; it has brought vividly to mind the importance of family to me as my own nuclear family dissolves. (In actuality, I find there is also an expansion, as the children bring back "significant others" and we move towards a larger collection of loosely connected adults.) It is not all bad, just difficult at times; writing this book and reading literature about families has helped me through this difficult transition. I think Hoffman has caught the process of family change so well:

> Families are notable examples of entities that change through leaps. The individuals making up a family are growing (at least partly) according to an internal biological design, but the larger groupings within the family, the subsystems and the generations, must endure major shifts in relation to each other.
>
> The task of family is to produce and train new sets of humans to be independent, form new families, and repeat the process, as the old set loses power, declines and dies. Family life is a multigenerational changing of the guard. And although this process is at times a smooth one, like the transitions of political parties in a democracy, it is more often fraught with danger and disruption.
>
> Most families do not leap to new integration with ease, and the transformations are by no means self-assured.[1]

My passion for families has carried over into my professional life and it is my unabashed opinion that if I can foster a greater concern for the family among

---

[1]Hoffman, L. (1981). *Foundations of family therapy.* New York: Basic Books, p. 160.

those professionals who work with the deaf child, we will be better able to help produce a generation of well functioning adults who happen to be deaf. Toward this end I want to encourage professionals to look at the family as an immense resource that can be used to work in the hearing-impaired child's interest.

My first professional encounter with the role of family in the management of hearing impairment occurred when, as a young audiologist, I saw an elderly woman who was brought to the clinic by her two daughters. Both daughters were very angry at their mother, who had refused so far to get a hearing aid, and they were very tired of shouting at her. I tested the woman and found that she did have a significant hearing loss, and while there were some auditory discrimination problems, she could probably benefit from wearing an aid. When I asked her why she refused to wear amplification, she told to me in private that she was afraid that if she had a hearing aid her daughters would call her on the phone and would no longer visit: she was much more afraid of being alone than of not hearing.

I dealt with this family by telling the children that their mother could only get limited help from amplification. If she wanted to get a hearing aid she would contact me but in the meantime they should not try to get her to wear an aid. This relieved the pressure on my client but it did not solve the family issue. I never heard from the family again. Looking at that clinical situation from a 25-year perspective, I wish dearly that I could have that family back. I now would feel comfortable in dealing with everyone's needs and, perhaps, if I had worked with the whole family, everyone could have gotten a win.

In 1965, having decided to gradually phase myself out of clinical audiology, which I was finding uncongenial, I started a parent-centered nursery for young hearing-impaired children. The program was conceived as a transition program for parents as they moved from diagnosis to entering the educational establishment. I served as facilitator of a parent support group which was a required component of the program and, as a result, I have found what has become for me a very satisfying life work.[2]

Now, with over 20 years of intimate relationships with many parents of deaf children, I often wonder in what dimension do I, as a parent of four "normal" children, differ from them; I have not found a single emotion that is unique to the parents I work with. There are two dimensions of parenting, however, that are different. For parents of hearing-impaired children there is a sense of sadness and of loss about their children that will never go away. They also take nothing for granted; savoring every gain, and rejoicing and celebrating the small, and sometimes large, victories that are part of working intensely with a disabled child. I am always struck by how much growth and joy can emerge from so much pain and suffering. Participating with parents so intimately has intensified my own parenting experience and has given me an opportunity to hone my skills; I owe the parents a great deal for allowing me

---

[2]Luterman, D. (1979). *Counseling parents of hearing impaired children.* Boston: Little, Brown and Co.

to share their experiences.

In this book I want to serve as a conduit to transmit and perhaps translate the family experience as I have seen it and worked with families over these years. I want to give the reader a feel for what it is like inside a family with a deaf child. This book is intended for professionals who are interested in intensifying their work with the families of hearing-impaired children. I have no doubt that much of the material in this book would be applicable to families in which there were disabilities other than deafness.

During the course of writing this book I have been delving into literature on the family, which I have found to be an immensely rich and still unmined lode of material that is quite relevant to our field. There is, however, very little research into families with disabled children. Most of the research has been on families of mentally retarded children, because the population is fairly large and can be easily specified as to the degree of handicap. There is an extreme paucity of data on families with deaf children; the studies can easily be counted on the fingers of both hands. I ardently hope that this book is rapidly rendered obsolete: that it becomes the stimulus for badly needed research. I have used the research from the other disabilities as well as what little does exist in deafness; I have come to the conclusion that there is very little that is unique to the families which have a deaf child as compared to those with any other disabled child. The issues seem to be the same. Of both necessity and choice, then, this book is written from a clinical and personal perspective.

What I have also wanted to do in this book is to have some of the families who have gone through the parent-centered program with me tell their stories. Many of them have remained my friends, and over the years I have watched them and their children grow. I have also watched them as they encountered the problems of managing transitions in the family life cycle, with the added complication of having a hearing-impaired child. Many of their problems and issues have been the same as mine.

In Chapters 2, 4, and 6 I have recorded in-depth interviews with three families, and scattered throughout the book are comments and observations that parents and other family members have shared with me over the years, and which I think are particularly relevant. I have made no attempt to make these parents representative of all families in any way; these are mainly middle-class families who are my friends and whose stories I want to tell.

I have not interviewed any deaf parents of deaf children as I am not facile in sign language and am uncomfortable working through interpreters when emotionally laden material is being discussed. My limited experience with deaf parents suggests that they respond differently than hearing parents. For example, a deaf husband and wife; awaiting the arrival of their first-born, were expecting the child to be deaf, and welcomed the deafness, "for it would have meant closer kinship in the family."[3] Clearly, the stresses in the deaf-parent families are very different from the stresses of hearing parents. The book

---

[3]Jacobs, L. (1980). *A deaf adult speaks out.* Washington, D.C.: Gallaudet Press.

documenting the experiences of deaf parents of deaf children needs to be written, but it will have to be written by someone else. In the same vein I did not interview any deaf children. I do not want to take attention away from the hearing member of the family, whose story I think is seldom heard. I prefer in this book to deal with the ripples rather than the stone and I want to keep the focus on the impact that the deaf child has on the hearing family members. However, each interview was sent back to the family with the suggestion that the deaf child read it and write a response to it if they wished. The child's responses, in those families which elected to have the hearing-impaired child react, may be found at the end of each chapter.

All the data in Chapters 2, 4, and 6 reported in this book were recorded by me during an interview with the family members. I then edited the material into its present form. I rearranged material so that it would read clearly and tried to eliminate some of the redundancy. In the course of working on those chapters I developed a profound respect for any novelist who writes dialogue.

For my first interview I nervously prepared a list of questions. I found, as I should have known beforehand, that the list was counterproductive: it tended to make the conversation stilted; I ceased to listen, sitting there desperately trying to think of my next question. Part way through the first interview I abandoned the list. What is reported in Chapter 2, 4, and 6 is the result of a somewhat edited, spontaneous interaction between me and the family members.

ACKNOWLEDGMENTS

I am always struck by how much support and help I need to write a book, and fortunately I have had considerable assistance on this one. I owe an enormous debt of gratitude to the families I call the "Wagners," the "Murphys," and the "Marshalls," who gave so willingly of their time and were so candid in describing their lives. I am also grateful to all those family members cited anonymously throughout the text who also shared themselves with me. Friends and colleagues such as Sue Colten and Mark Ross read parts of the manuscript and gave generously of their time and criticism. Daniel Ling, in addition to writing the foreword, gave many helpful editorial suggestions. Nathaniel Knight and Bob Sullivan showed an uncanny knack in finding obscure references for me. Both of them had the tenacity and patience of saints in locating and acquiring needed books. Brian McCarthy had the incredible ability to read my handwriting and translate my scribbles into readable copy. He always bent to the task cheerfully and accomplished it with dispatch. I am grateful to them all.

CHAPTER 1

Family in Theory

The origin of clinical work with families, like that of most innovations, cannot be attributed to any one person; instead, it seems to have developed fairly spontaneously in the 1950s and 1960s from the work of disparate clinicians. Satir, Ackerman, Jackson, and Whitaker were among the originators of the current thinking about families and their role in the development of pathology in individuals (Hoffman, 1981). All of these clinicians, trained in individual therapy, often found that the gains made in therapy were lost once the individuals went back into their families. For example, Jackson found that a young, hospitalized man he was working with was perfectly rational in individual therapy but became highly "schizophrenic" shortly after his mother visited him. It was a bold step for these clinicians to work with the whole family and to examine the pathology embedded within the family structure; but, from this step came the origins of family therapy and the notion of the family as a system.

The most fundamental concept in family systems theory is that all the components of the system are interdependent. That is, every member of the family affects every other member and change in one member causes changes in all other members. For the family therapist, there is no such thing as individual therapy. Any attempt to change one member of the family will have an impact on the whole family.

A family can be compared to an engine in which there is a reciprocal arrangement among the various components. Where an emotionally ill person has been identified, the family therapists see

1

this as a design "flaw" in the engine. To merely repair the broken "part" without changing the structural relationships in the family "engine" is very often useless, because the individual component is not strong enough to overcome the defective architecture of the family. R. D. Laing commented that schizophrenia is a rational response to an impossible situation.

Consequently, family therapists take the whole engine into therapy and, by working with the system, try to create a healthy, functioning environment in which each component has space to grow. I know, for example, a child psychologist who does not see children; he sees only the parents, because he finds that when the parents' problems are cleared up, the child's behavior also improves. This notion, whether we realize it or not, is the basis of early intervention programs, where we work closely with families in order to create a healthy environment for the deaf child. The underlying assumption is that "If you take good care of the family, the child will do well."

In our field, essentially, we work with normal families who are under a great deal of stress because they include a hearing-impaired child. Family therapists tend to work with families in distress and unable to function. Nevertheless, many of the concepts developed by the family therapists are very relevant to work with deafness and with families with a disabled child. In this chapter, I discuss concepts from the family therapy literature that are particularly relevant to professionals who work with families that include a disabled child.[1]

THE FAMILY AS SYSTEM

All family members are connected to one another, and any behavior or change in behavior of one member affects all members. This includes members of the parents' families of origin (the grandparents) and is not limited to the nuclear family. The general systems theory says that each variable in any system interacts with the other variables so thoroughly that cause and effect cannot be separated. This notion implies that, when a deaf child is born into a family, to some extent, everybody is "deaf."

An important component of the system effect is the notion of triangulation; in fact, the family system can be viewed as a series of

---

[1]The discussion of some of the concepts underlying family theory and family therapy, of necessity, is simplified. The interested reader is referred to the excellent text *Foundations of Family Therapy* by Hoffman (New York: Basic Books, 1981).

interlocking triangles. Triangulation is a process, occuring in all families and in all social groups, in which twosomes form to the exclusion of a third. The basic triangle in families is between both parents and the child. The interaction among all three is highly complex. For example, Minuchin (1974), the family therapist who developed the concept of triangulation, worked closely with families in which a child was anorexic. In his research, he frequently found a similar pattern of interaction among the parents with their children. In the initial lunch session, a standard feature of Minuchin's treatment, he often found one authoritarian parent who tried to force the child to eat, while the other parent pulled back and gave way in an attempt to calm the child and soften the effect. The child was caught in a classic dilemma: If she[2] ate she was supporting one parent against the other; if she didn't she would be forming a coalition with the other. In addition, the action escalated so that she was pulled harder and harder in both directions at the same time.

In many families, Minuchin found that the parents' concern for the child's anorexia masked issues in their own relationship. In fact, it often appeared that the child was holding the parents' marriage together through her anorectic symptoms. Therapeutic interventions based on Minuchin's notions that a child's symptoms are linked to parental conflict have been unusually successful (Hoffman, 1981). The goal of Minuchin's therapy is a structural one: to dislodge the child from a position between the parents and to help the parents deal more directly with their own problems. When this is done, the child can give up her anorexia.

A similar process occurs very frequently in families with a deaf child. Mendelsohn and Rozek (1983) feel that the "intrinsic characteristics of the deafness and the caretaking process lend themselves to the child being easily triangulated into anxious or conflictual areas in the family life. The disability puts the child into focus more easily because of the need for more attention and care."

The notion of triangulation has profound implications for all professionals working with families containing a deaf child. For example, in those families in which the father is distant, which is fairly common, programs usually try to strengthen the father-child bond by seducing the father into involvement with the program. A recent conference of educators of the hearing impaired had a session devoted entirely to "Involving Fathers in Home Intervention." Among the suggestions developed were to establish rapport with the father early;

---

[2]I use the pronoun *she* because anorexia is most common in females.

to take time to write or leave a note for the father; to make a specific phone call to him; to include the father in regularly scheduled visits; to give the father assignments; and, of course, to reinforce the father for his good work (Ski Hi Communicative Disorder Institute, 1985) I think these strategies will work nicely in some families; that is, families in which the father is timid about involving himself with his child. This is especially true with first time fathers of very young children. It must be kept in mind that, when you attempt to change the father-child bond, you will also alter the mother-child and the mother-father relationships: You cannot tinker with one part of the triangle without altering the other parts.

Moreover, many times, techniques to attract the father fail or do so only momentarily, with the father soon resuming his distant behavior. Invariably, the professional starts searching for another gimmick to attract the father or enters into a subtle coalition with the mother, thus forming another triangle, which further excludes and alienates the father. Family system theory tells us that we can affect the father-child relationship by working with the mother-child relationship or the husband-wife relationship. Very often, the cause of the father's distancing may lie within the mother-child dyad or the marital relationship. In fact, when one begins to look at the mother-child relationship in families with distant fathers, one invariably finds mothers who are bonded very closely with their child and who really do not want the father to take an active part, despite their protestation to the contrary. Many of these mothers have unresolved feelings of guilt and feel that "repairing the damage" is their responsibility. One also frequently sees mothers who get a great deal of reward and satisfaction from working with their child. For many mothers, the deaf child becomes a means of realizing their self-worth. They thoroughly enjoy working with their child and very often do not leave much room for the fathers.

Also, there are wives who simply need a club to wield over their husbands and prefer to complain about them. In families such as these, attempts to coax the father to participate will fail, and it is always poor family management for the therapist or teacher to enter into an unholy alliance with the mother against the father.

One needs also to look at another leg of the triangle. A considerable body of research indicates that the father's relationship with his wife strongly influences the mother-child relationship. The husband/father's emotional support of the wife/mother enhances the mother's capacity to meet the affectional and caregiving needs of the infant; conversely, in families where there is an emotionally distant husband, there tends to be an emotionally distant mother (Pedersen, 1976).

Very often, most people's view of the family is that the parents, have a paramount influence over the child. What is overlooked, but which systems theory would fully support, is that the child's behavior equally influences the parents' behavior. There is a bidirectional flow of effect and, as we shall see, perceived "success" by the parents in terms of their expectations for the child leads to changes in their behavior. 'Successful'' children are less restricted by parents, while less successful children are restricted further.

FAMILY HOMEOSTASIS

As in any system, families always will seek to maintain a sense of order, balance, and continuity in their family life. This means that families tend to resist change, although they must accommodate change as they go through their life cycle. On the simplest level, for example, when a parent is away on a business trip for a few days then returns to the family, there is always a period of adjustment. While the parent is gone, all other members of the family have to fill parts of that role and assume additional responsibilities in order for the family to continue to function. Some functions can be on hold but others have to be taken over. When the parent returns, the family must readjust and a child could quite rightly accuses the parent of ordering him or her about to reestablish the role as parent. This conflict results from the parent's need to reestablish the previous homeostasis and again find a place in the family.

Homeostasis also explains why when children leave the family, as when they go to college, they can never return, nor should they, in quite the same way. They have become part of another system that alters them, and their leaving the family alters the family, so it is no longer the same unit that the child left. In fact, the child becomes a "spare part" and is not necessary to the functioning of the family. One sees this very often in families in which there are deaf parents and a hearing child. The deaf parents often feel that they have to rely on the hearing child to function and the child readily accepts this role. When the hearing child does leave, usually with much difficulty, the parents do not necessarily fall apart but find other ways of coping. This notion is developed very well in Greenberg's novel, In This Sign (1970).

The drive to maintain homeostasis is seen especially at diagnosis, when parents find it very hard to accept their child as being disabled. Having a deaf child means also that the family will have to change, that everyone will now have to respond differently, and that new demands will be placed on the family structure. This challenge to homeostatis is invariably met with resistance.

All change, whether it be positive or negative, involves stress because it challenges homeostatis. In addition, there is no growth without some stress. The problem that families must resolve is how to maintain stability in the face of the normal changes that occur as families go through the life cycle. For our purposes, we need to explore how families maintain balance in the face of the severe crisis and stress generated by having a child who is deaf.

FAMILY PARADIGM

One notion of how families cope with crises is the idea of the family paradigm. A paradigm is a framework of thought, a scheme for understanding and explaining certain aspects of reality. The notion of paradigm and paradigm shift, as a means of understanding the growth and change in science, was first introduced by Kuhn in *The Structure of Scientific Revolution* (1974). Kuhn sees scientists as a quasi-social group, whose behavior is shaped by a set of assumptions, or a paradigm, about the natural world. As scientists begin to accumulate new pieces of data that do not fit into the explanation afforded by the prevailing paradigm, conflict ensues in the scientific community. At some point, a change in perspective or a paradigmatic shift occurs through the efforts of a scientist who looks at the universe in a startlingly different way; for example, Einstein's special theory of relativity formed the new paradigm that superseded Newtonian physics and Copernicus' heliocentric view of the planets sharply contrasted with the prevailing geocentric view. Shift is not accomplished without stress; in order for the new perspective to be accepted, the old one must be discarded, which often causes pain. At first, the new may be greeted with skepticism and, sometimes, with outright hostility. Very often, it is the next generation of scientists who accept the new paradigm, until that paradigm is eventually replaced by still another paradigmatic shift.

Kuhn also points out that the paradigmatic shift occurs suddenly. It is rarely incremental but is a new way of looking at things. Although Kuhn was writing about science, the notion of paradigm and paradigmatic shift have been widely adopted by other professions. By naming this recognizable phenomenon, Kuhn has made us aware of how change is accomplished; that is, by a series of paradigmatic shifts that generally are first met by resistance.

Reiss (1981) adapted the notion of paradigm and paradigmatic shift to families. According to Reiss, each individual develops his or her own personal paradigm; this is a central organizer of viewing the world, composed of constructs, expectations, and fantasies of the social world, and becomes a personal explanatory system. When two or more people develop an intimate relationship, they both must reconcile their personal paradigms to form a family paradigm. Dissolutions of families can result from the incompatibility of the personal paradigms.

This is not to say that families cannot have fights. Reiss cites the example of a husband and wife who have a shouting match because their child's toys were left on the lawn. Despite the argument both parents share a belief system about the value of neighbors' opinions and both feel that an argument is won by the person who shouts the loudest. Divorces, I think, are more likely in families in which one member always picks up the toys and never fights.

Growth for both individuals and families can be seen as a series of tests to a prevailing paradigm, and change results from the shift in paradigm. Stress becomes the impetus for causing paradigm shift. This notion becomes very valuable when looking at the family under stress because of a hearing-impaired, or otherwise disabled, child. Any time there is change within the family there will be challenge to the prevailing paradigm, as, for example, when a child is moved from an oral program to a total communication program. However, the greatest stress on the family occurs at the diagnosis and shortly thereafter, when a whole new paradigm for the family has to be established. They are now a "deaf family" and they must somehow deal with this new reality. Another serious crisis time for the family occurs when the hearing-impaired child needs to leave and the parents need to let go. This also requires a severe paradigmatic shift.

Growth in all healthy families can be seen as a process of discarding old paradigms and replacing them with more useful ones. Unhealthy families try to maintain the old paradigm in the face of a new reality. The process of working with families of a handicapped child can be seen as one of helping them construct new and useful paradigms.

THE OPTIMAL FAMILY

Family therapists, by definition, are almost invariably working with disordered families. These are not necessarily the families seen in educational programs for the deaf. Both family therapists and professionals working with families having a disabled child need a vision of an optimal family. In other words, what are we working toward with the families we encounter? There are several different models of the optimal family (Beavers & Voeller; Epstein, Bishop, & Baldwin, 1982; Olson, Russell, & Sprenkle, 1983). All seem to agree that the healthy family would have the following characteristics:

1. *Communication among all members is clear and direct.* In an optimal family there is no hesitation or holding back, no talking around an issue. Comments are always directed to the person for whom they are intended. Talking is efficient and straightforward. Messages are congruent, containing both content and feeling. There is empathy and humor in the communications among family members.

2. *Roles and responsibilities are clearly delineated, and the family allows for flexibility in role allocation.* An optimal family must have clear boundaries. There must be a clear intergenerational boundary as well as a sibling boundary. The parents must have clear authority. At the same time, the family must allow flexibility in roles to accommodate change. There must be a basis and structure for negotiation. The children's responsibilities need to alter as they grow, and responsibilities need to be renegotiated periodically. Optimal families allow for the change in roles as needed to maintain a well functioning unit.

3. *The family members accept limits for the resolution of conflict.* Conflict is ever present in families. Healthy families resolve conflict at an individual or family level. They do not avoid or deny conflict. Individual needs are always considered in attempting a resolution of any dispute, and there are face-saving mechanisms, too.

4. *Intimacy is prevalent and is a function of frequent, equal-powered transactions.* One of the basic functions of family is to provide intimacy. Human beings need environments where there is closeness and caring. An optimal family provides intimacy while also respecting the need for space and distance. Optimal families are cohesive without being enmeshed.

5. *There is a healthy balance between change and the maintenance of stability.* Families must change to accommodate the life cycle and life's vicissitudes, such as having a deaf child, the death of parents, or sometimes social or economic catastrophe. Optimal families are able to make the necessary changes while maintaining stability; the stress of the change is accommodated and the family makes the necessary alterations.

For Beavers and Voeller (1983), the optimal family "tolerates well its evolution through time, actually encouraging its own demise as a tightly knit group. In its later stages of development, it becomes a loosely connected, lovingly respectful group of equal adults with grandchildren to raise. Each individual knows that he or she needs the family, and this knowledge assists capable, comfortable negotiation."

Optimal families should produce optimal hearing-impaired children and adults, and our goal as professionals is to help the family to achieve its potential by enhancing the characteristics of optimal families.

Armed with these notions of family systems, triangulation, homeostasis, paradigm, and optimal functioning, let us look at some families.

REFERENCES

Beavers, R., & Voeller, M. (1983). Comparing and contrasting the Olson Circumplex Model with the Beavers Systems Model. *Family Process, 22,* 85–98.

Epstein, N., Bishop, D., & Baldwin, L. (1982). McMaster Model of family functioning: A view of the normal family. In Fromm Walsh (Ed.), *Normal family process.* New York: Guilford Press.

Greenberg, J. (1970). *In this sign.* New York: Holt, Rinehart and Winston.

Hoffman, L. (1981). *Foundations of family therapy.* New York: Basic Books.

Kuhn, T. (1974). *The structure of scientific revolutions.* Chicago: The University of Chicago Press.

Mendelsohn, M., & Rozek, F. (1983). Denying disability: The case of deafness. *Family Systems Medicine, I* (2), 37–47.

Minuchin, S. (1974). *Families and family therapy.* Cambridge, MA: Harvard University Press.

Olson, D., Russell, C., & Sprenkle, D. (1983). Circumflex Model of marital and family systems: VI. Theoretical update. *Family Process, 22,* 69–83.

Pedersen, F. (1976). Does research on children reared in father absent families yield information on father influences. *Family Coordinator, 25,* 459–463.

Reiss, D. (1981). *The family's construction of reality.* Cambridge, MA: Harvard University Press.

Ski*Hi Communicative Disorder Institute (1985). National Summer Conference, Utah State University.

CHAPTER 2

Family in Practice:
The Wagners

Bill and Lydia Wagner have three children: Laura, Kate, and Conrad. The oldest, Laura, 22, currently attends a private university in Massachusetts that is her father's alma mater. Laura is profoundly deaf. Kate and Conrad are younger. Bill is a successful businessman and Lydia, who was formerly a teacher, has spent most of the child-rearing years as a housewife. As the children left the home, she has begun to work outside.

D.L.: Can you tell me some of your experiences with Laura?

Lydia: Laura was diagnosed at 8 months of age. I had German measles during the rubella epidemic. She was diagnosed by her grandfather, who was living with us. He would go into her room in the morning and she would be very startled when she saw him. Knowing that I had German measles, she had been through extensive testing, but nobody suspected hearing loss. After she was diagnosed, we spent a short period of time in a program in a fire station. We went from there to the Emerson program for two years. And after that, we went to a nursery for hearing children and we were getting private tutoring for her from a teacher of the deaf. Then, we went into a day program for deaf children in a public school. We spent two years there, and then we made a big move. It was apparent that Laura wasn't getting what she needed, so we put her in a residential school for the deaf, where she stayed from age 7 to age 11. From there, she was mainstreamed into a small, private girls school. Now, she is a senior in college, and she just missed the Dean's List.

Bill: She has had a tutor and a notetaker in her college classes, and she had tutors ever since she left the school for the deaf.

Lydia: And this year, at college, she has requested an interpreter. We don't know how necessary that was, but she got that on her own.

The worst part of the story for me begins before she was diagnosed because I knew I had German measles. From the 13th week on, I wondered what would happen. It was something I had no control over. And from the 13th week of pregnancy until she was delivered probably was the worst part, as far as I was concerned. There was so much stress—a terrible feeling of lack of control.

Bill: I remember a lot of discussion after Laura was born about having another child right away. We really didn't know what was the cause, just here was a defective child. We needed to produce a normal child. There is only 16 months difference between Laura's birth and Kate's. The deafness intensified the inadequacies we felt and I wondered whether my next child would be defective, too.

Lydia: I remember that Kate had breathing problems and we were very worried about her. Conrad had head trauma problems. All three children had very difficult infancies.

Bill: I worried a lot about the younger children because of the problem with Laura.

Lydia: Obviously, I was more cautious in my later pregnancies. Remember when I was pregnant with Conrad; you had cold sores and your mother came and took care of you and I moved out of the house? When Kate was born, I remember Bill and me sitting outside her door and listening to her babble. It was wonderful! She would talk to herself at night before falling asleep. I thought it was a miracle.

I think being the oldest child made Laura more independent. I think she would have been my baby for the rest of her life if she was the youngest. With Kate and Conrad right behind, I couldn't afford to let her be dependent. I remember sitting in the car with Kate and sending Laura into the store to get something, not knowing if she could make herelf understood. We pushed her and encouraged her. It was hard to take her to birthday parties and to do all kinds of things. Maybe if she was the youngest, I would have softened the atmosphere for her more.

D.L.: The deafness sure complicated your child rearing.

Lydia: Yes. I'm always aware that I don't know how Laura feels. Not that anybody knows how anybody else feels. I can imagine more clearly how one of my other kids feels in a situation, but I really don't know what makes Laura feel tense and stressful. I've never experienced her problems. So that's tough on a mother. I just didn't know what she was thinking, how she was feeling, but she had lots of guts, which was great.

D.L.: You have made a lot of changes. How did you two make those decisions?

Bill: I think most things become very apparent if you look around a bit; one thing is clearly better than the other or it is the only thing available. There really were never too many conflicts, other than going to the school for the deaf.

Lydia: I remember when we made that decision because I visited a lot at the day class and I was a teacher. I would come home and say to Bill, "I don't think she is getting what she needs."
    Many times I would feed Bill the information. I was never afraid to make changes. I don't think those two years in the day class were wasted. Those years were important; I couldn't have sent her away then.

Bill: She would give me the information and we made many moves, but we didn't have any internal friction over any of them.

Lydia: No. Once we made the decision, you always had the guts to say the difficult things, like telling the educators at the school for the deaf that we would only be there for a little while.

D.L.: So he would be the front man and you would be behind the scenes gathering the data?

Bill: Yes, it seemed that way.

D.L.: How else did you divide your roles?

Lydia: I don't know. It sort of evolved.

Bill: I don't think it evolved. Lydia had the ball all of the time. The only thing I contributed—and it was a hard thing— many times when you were down I did little things. I can remember getting up in the morning and giving Laura some speech lessons, and just that little was enough to keep Lydia going.

Lydia: We got a lot of support from Bill's parents, who would come and babysit so we could go away for a weekend. We did that almost every six weeks. And Bill's father also would drive once a week to pick up Laura at the school for the deaf. That was a big help. It was over a hundred miles each way and we had to do it twice a week. They would do one trip for us. My father used to take care of Kate when I went to the nursery. It would have been so difficult if we were in a different part of the country. There were so many people involved. The family was a big help.

Bill: I think our involvement with the parent association was a big help. We got into the political issue and then it became part of our social life. They became our good friends and that helped both of us.

D.L.: What did you do in the process, Bill?

Bill: Not a whole lot. Lydia did most of the work, and I think the support came from two ways. Sometimes the group helped us with Laura and we got excited as a couple about what we were trying to do for deafness in general.

Lydia: Plus you had the attitude in life definitely that, of course, it can be done. I can remember in the parents' association when we were trying to get programs started you would always say "Don't worry about that. The money will always come. Just decide what you want." I remember lying in bed thinking one morning how glad I was that you were there, and that I was not alone.

Bill: It's hard for a man. He doesn't know his child very well because he's working and his wife is home. I always felt very awkward. But that was always a tinderbox. I guess I knew enough to help out.

Lydia: I remember we had the table in our room and you used to work with her when I was still in bed.

D.L.: It sounds like Laura's deafness permeated your whole life.

Lydia: Yes, it sure did. So many of our friends were associated with deafness.

Bill: It was either that or the marriages break up. It was such a big job and never seems to end. And I think people get frightened. It was one of those things where you walk the center of the line. We were able to use the people we met as support for us, whereas other people didn't invest so much time and effort and it drove them apart.

D.L.: Has Laura's deafness strengthened your marriage?

Lydia: We endured. It's hard to say. I think it has certainly given us something very strong that we can look back on and say we did a good job at, that we really worked together. And we can be proud of that. I don't know if it strengthened our marriage; it was certainly a lot of stress, which we could have done without, and it gave us less fun time together. There were so many other stresses, too. Bill was building his business, then my mother died and my father came to live with us.

Bill: It turned the marriage into a working marriage right away. Lydia was pregnant only three months after we were married, and we never really relaxed.

Lydia: We never really chose to relax—that's for sure—not until recently. Laura's deafness has not been a big issue for a long time now.

Bill: She has been extraordinarily independent, which took off the stress. I began to relax when she was mainstreamed and we got the tutor and I began to see that she was going to make it. The tutor was a big help.

D.L.: Did you see any stress on Kate and Conrad?
Lydia: Oh, yeah. When Laura went to the residential school for the deaf we all really were upset. The kids couldn't have a normal sibling relationship. We all had the feeling, subconsciously, that we couldn't push Laura too far. It was tough.

Bill: Laura realized her limitations and she reacted violently. The other kids tiptoed, literally, in terms of their relationship with her. Laura was the one to be served. Everybody in the whole family knew that.

Lydia: And she let you know that, too. Not that she demanded more, but there was so much that she didn't understand. She was very feisty. Sometimes I thought the roof would fall in because she would bang the doors so hard.

Bill: Loads of frustration. In talking, she did not get what was said and we had to repeat everything. It was not enjoyable. There was so much frustration. The first time we knew what a normal family was like was when she went away to school and we could have a normal dinner conversation. When she wasn't there, the house ran a lot smoother.

Lydia: It was so hard to send her away. It was awful. I remember at that time the kindness of so many people. The sensitivity of Bill's father—the first week we sent Laura away he came to visit us every night. He just stopped in and it was very pleasant. He really touched me. It was a wonderful thing because people knew how hard it was to send her away.

The first weekend we went to pick her up she cried when she saw us because she didn't like the peas and carrots. And I thought it was more than the peas and carrots she didn't like. It was hard. It was a break from the family. I remember when she came home on the weekend she would run up to her room to see what was touched. She was a witch.

It did give Laura some deaf friends. It gave her a network that she still needs. Even now, she keeps in touch with those friends.

D.L.: I see the stresses in the family. Do you see any positives?

Lydia: She made me stretch, tremendously. I feel a tremendous sense of integrity from my relationship with her. I worked really hard. There are so many payoffs now. She is comfortable with herself and she is successful.

Bill: She helped the other kids—Conrad's language development was so much better because Lydia kept putting the language in for Laura.

Lydia: I learned a lot about language and I had a lot of fun with Laura. I feel good about myself. I never thought I could have worked this hard on a task. I feel a sense of authenticity. She was the biggest job of my life, definitely, and I did a good job with her, and I can live well with that. There was so much stress in having Laura, but I am definitely the better for it. I never knew I had so much drive and self-control and all kinds of things. As far as the other kids, I think they are sensitive and patient. I think we have a nice family sense.

D.L.: It seems like she was at times a unifying force in the family. Even though she was stressful.

Bill: At the beginning at least, it was not unifying. I think it was more a period that was successfully completed. I don't think there was much joy in it.

Lydia: Except for the support. I am very touched when I think back on all the support we received from friends. And the relationships that developed because of Laura, I value very highly. That's a big positive.

Bill: We also got further into feelings and emotions. I don't know if we would have gotten into it if we had three normal kids. I'm sort of insensitive and I wouldn't have gotten into these to any extent. The whole tenor of the past 20 years has been of feelings and sensitivities. She broadened me out. I learned more acceptance. I was confused at the first part. The Emerson program was really the keystone. We entered the program at a very vulnerable time but also a very fertile time. There is no question about it. We needed some direction, and we got it.

Lydia: We got confidence that we could do it, and that we could bump her around and make changes, and that we were not fragile. We got the confidence that we knew, once we began to think, that we knew more than the educators.

Bill: That and when you [D.L.] brought together some other couples, I think the group therapy and talking about feelings and inadequacies was very helpful. I didn't know much about that stuff at the time, but it really was a good thing, being thrown together with other people who had a similar problem. Everybody would tell their story and you didn't feel so alone.

Lydia: There was a tremendous bond among the members of the group. It was so special. I remember getting phone calls from people who moved out-of-state after the program. After two sentences, we were right down to what was real. Having a handicapped child first, I found that I had so little in common with my friends who were having their first babies. I had nothing in common with them, and sometimes I'd get angry with them if they were complaining about something. The group was just tremendous.
   They were people who could rejoice with us and be sad with us. I find it hard to socialize with my friends.

D.L.: It sounds like Laura helped you get your priorities squared away.

Lydia: Yeah, she did, fast, and that's good. We are grateful to her for that. Anyway, the time has gone quickly. The one thing we didn't do was live in the present. That was the one thing we didn't do enough of. There was always one more goal, one more word to be learned. There was always so much to be done. That is probably what we are going to do now, live more in the present.

Bill: Yeah. The goals drove us. We accepted our roles and we lost a lot of fun. We treated it as work. This might have been culture or religion or it might have been our personalities.

D.L.: This was a cross to bear?

Bill: Yeah, it could have been our cross to bear, although it was a little more human than a cross. It was our kid. And it was seeing how well we could do for our child. But you know it was an unending job. It wasn't any 8 to 5. We were instructing the kid twenty-four hours a day. And, you could run yourself out of energy.

Lydia: It also looked like forever in the future. That was the thing. It was such a huge problem, to bear so much. What also helped us so much was Laura's success and our economic means; if there was anything we felt we needed, we could do it.

Bill: The greatest thing she had was her social nature. She would always go up to talk to people. She has always been that way. I don't think it's because of her deafness. She knows the president of the college and goes to see him. She always saw herself as having worth, and because of that, she didn't have to hang back. Some of it is innate and some of it is from the programs she has been in.

My biggest fear of the future is that Laura will fall through the slats. She doesn't have enough deaf friends who are doing what she does; she is somewhat isolated from the deaf community. She goes to some deaf groups, and they don't believe that she is deaf. That's a great worry. The residential school gave her a deaf identity and some deaf friends.

Her closest friends are still her deaf friends. She wants to marry a hard-of-hearing boy. We are at an interesting point. She is going to start interviewing for a job. So we set her up with a job counselor. We've always felt that Laura should get a job in an objective area like mathematics or computers. She's good at them, but Laura has not seen this.

Lydia: She wants to work much more with people.

Bill: But we have some concerns. I think it's very important for her self-esteem that she get a job and start working. You know, I'm not too frightened about that. She's gone over so many big hurdles. Not using the telephone and finding a job is going to a big one, but she'll get over it. I've had great fears for Laura, you know; first of all because of her deafness: getting hit by cars and things like that. But then, because of her naiveté: drugs and things like this. Loads of concerns en route. Some of the guys she has dated! It's probably good for us that a lot of this happened away from our house.

The thing that bothers us is that she is socially immature and that can get you into a lot of trouble. She's not street smart but she's learned a lot. She doesn't understand some basic things. She throws around words and she seems to understand some things so well, but doesn't understand some things that sixth graders know. All of her victories have come at a price.

D.L.: It seems you paid a price, too. Was it worth it?

Lydia: Yes. I really like her. I was the one who had the most difficulty with her and we have a good relationship now. I like her and I admire her a lot. She has good instincts.

Bill: It's been worth it. But it's worth it a lot more in retrospect. Going through it was very hard.

Lydia: It wasn't just Laura. It was also that Bill was building a business and coming home exhausted.

D.L.: What role did Poppa [Lydia's father] play?

Lydia: He always had time for the kids. Even when we didn't. He gave the kids those little extras that I didn't, like taking them to the dump and bringing back more things than they dropped off. He was always helping fix things or looking for a part of a toy. He gave them a tremendous amount of himself. He adored Laura and he was a real support to the kids. I learned early that I couldn't really share my fears with Poppa because he had already lived his life and had his share of problems. And I didn't think it was his place to support me emtionally, other than the ways he was doing. He had a wonderful disposition. He knew which way the kids liked things and he pleased them. He gave them a lot of time.

Bill: It was nice that they had someone like Poppa who wasn't their parent or their teacher. Someone that they could just enjoy.

D.L.: So he filled some of those gaps that you were missing.

Lydia: Yes, definitely.

Bill: Yes. But that also put some strains on our marriage.

Lydia: Yeah, we were never alone.

Bill: We were married, and then I guess you became pregnant and then your mother died.

Lydia: The night I broke out with German measles.

Bill: Your father couldn't really carry on by himself so we had him with us eight months after we got married. And we had him with us for 17 years.

Lydia: So it is all a tradeoff, right?

D.L.: So this the first time in your life that you have been alone together.

Lydia: Yeah. It's great. It's fantastic.

Bill: Then, Conrad went off to college. The kids call and ask if we miss them. I tell them ''don't hurry home.''

D.L.: So there is a life after deafness?

Bill and Lydia: Yeah.

Kate, age 21, is a junior in a premed program at a university not far from her parent's home. Conrad, age 19, is a freshman English major at the same university as Kate. This interview was conducted at a different time and place from that with their parents.

D.L.: Can you recall when you became aware that your sister was deaf?

Kate: There was no sharp demarcation. We just knew that some people wore hearing aids and that others did not. It was not a conscious thing.

Conrad: The first thing I can remember, I was in kindergarten and we were doing little papers asking Santa Claus what we wanted for Christmas and I remember asking that Laura be un-deaf so that was my first realization that Laura was deaf, although, of course, I did not know what deaf meant. I guess I must have known that deaf was something bad.

Kate: We said the word *deaf* a lot at home and I can remember not knowing what the word meant and going to school and having the other kids not pronounce it right. Have you noticed how the other kids said *death* instead of *deaf*? I can remember thinking that I knew something about it and I should correct them.

Conrad: It always seemed so normal to us to have Laura deaf. You need somebody else to come in and get the perspective, that there was something different about us.

Kate: We knew something was wrong because she didn't go to school with us. She was away at school and she only came home at weekends.

D.L.: Did you ever get to resent Laura's deafness?

Kate: No. We all went to different schools and I think Mom and Dad were very much aware that it could be a lopsided equation and they really did a great job with us. Because it seemed like even when we had to make extra time in conversation for her, it did not seem so bad.

Conrad: It might have been worse if there was just one other kid. I think the fact that we had two others helped a little bit. Aside from the extra attention she got and how hard it was in conversation, I don't remember that she monopolized Mom or Dad.

Kate: No. It really didn't matter. I think some of that was that we didn't realize the amount of energy that was put into it. I never realized it. It's an amazing thing now. They still like each other! They are still married. And, they still had time to make us feel that we were no less important than Laura. Not only do you realize it now about them, but you realize it about Laura, what a phenomenal thing that is. . . . You sort of feel responsible for that because of all the effort Mom and Dad and Laura put into it. You know in conversation or something about deafness or about the handicapped, I feel responsible to say something.

Conrad: Yes. You really do. You can't sit back. You feel that you have to mention it. That's probably because Mom and Dad did such a good job that we don't reject it but feel responsible.

D.L.: How did they make you part of it?

Kate: I remember the blackboard. In the kitchen, we had the blackboard and the three of us always ate together; and if there was a word or something that Laura didn't know, we could have the opportunity, could go and write it down, and we were getting just as much attention as she was. And she is learning the word or whatever.

Conrad: We really loved doing it. I can remember it made you feel a little bit big being able to teach your older sister something.

Kate: Yes. It was good for everybody. Mom could see her two kids, and you can feel a little inflated that you knew the word and Laura can learn something new. It was all done in a good environment. The tone was good. I don't know how they did that.

D.L.: Can you see any drawbacks and negatives in this?

Kate: It's frustrating. You have to repeat words and things and you get frustrated . . . and the worst thing you can do, which is what we always used to do, is to say, ''Forget it.'' She used to get so frustrated, because who wants to hear ''Forget it'? That's such a negative thing. But you get so frustrated repeating the word and repeating the word, that you think it is just not worth saying, but you realize that you have to be very patient.

Conrad: Yeah, it was negative because you always feel a bit of guilt and there was always some incredible responsibility to keep telling her the word. I always had this overblown sense that I had to keep following through, otherwise, I would feel guilty. That was negative. We had the overblown sense that we had to include her in everything. When, to be a normal person, sometimes you're not included. You know what I mean?

D.L.: Yes. Sometimes she was a pain in the neck and you felt guilty for feeling that.

Conrad: Right. So I'd feel bad because she's deaf and this is what I have to do. This was part of our upbringing, to always include her in everything.

Kate: It was very hard because it is very bad to feel like you were withholding something from someone else.

Conrad: I hated introducing kids to her. It was a stressful thing for me. I would bring friends over to the house, I would have to explain how my sister was deaf, and I didn't know how the other kid would react to Laura.

Kate: You had to have a lot of trust or faith in your friends.

D.L.: There was a part of you that was a little bit ashamed that you had a deaf sister.

Conrad: Yeah. I won't lie and say that all my friends were understanding. Some kids absolutely don't understand.

Kate: That's the scary thing because by just bringing somebody home, you had to confront someone with something they would have to deal with, and you don't know how they are going to deal with it. It's like a risk; I guess you just learn quickly some people just are not going to understand. You're the deaf person's sister.

D.L.: It must have been hard as a young child.

Conrad: It's still pretty hard now. The interaction, too, wears you out. It's tiring. It shouldn't be tiring, but it is.

D.L.: It takes so much effort to communicate.

Conrad: It takes less then it did, but it still takes a lot of effort.

Kate: You think of a family and you think everything is always happy from the start. There is something that is just very different. Like, all of a sudden, you learn that not everyone hears in the world. That is something that you probably learn very much later.

D.L.: You both had to learn it very early.

Kate: Not everyone hears. What does that mean? I have always heard. It's a very strange thing to know so quickly.

D.L.: And you find yourself wishing that you had a normal family like everybody else.

Kate: Yeah. That's a harsh thing to learn about the world—some people don't see, some people don't hear—when you are that little.

Conrad: I think you gotta bring Poppa into the picture.

Kate: I think Poppa made it seem different. Not only do you have a sister who can't hear, but this old person who is living with you. So, all of a sudden, this ideal conception of a family as being two people who are older and young people who are all the same; only we were not all the same. It was just very different.

D.L.: So there were two people in your family who didn't fit in.

Kate: I can remember doing percentages and thinking that two out of 6 of us wear hearing aids. That's 33 percent. I can rememeber that very distinctly . . . It's usually so routine, hearing aids etc., but every once in a while I hear something very good, and I can't even conceptualize that she can't hear that. That music will never make sense to her. That happens fairly frequently when you are really enjoying something. You can see her personality and how she tries so hard, and you ask why wasn't I the deaf one?

  ◢ I certainly don't merit it. It's luck. It's all luck. I think that's a family message, too. Not only luck in relationship to the deafness, but luck that you were born where you are. What's Mom always saying? Like you could have been born anywhere.

Conrad: Yeah. She keeps saying something that always makes me feel a little bit bad. 'It's only an accident of birth.''

Kate: That statement makes you feel very empty, just in the way when you listen to the music and try to conceptualize her not hearing, you feel very empty.

Conrad: It sure shoots out the legs from us a little bit, too, because we'd feel like, you know, we'd be in this nice house and we'd feel good that we sort of deserved it and then she'd come along and say, ''You are just here because it is an accident of birth.''

D.L.: It makes you feel very vulnerable, doesn't it?

Kate: Yes, very empty. And you feel as though you should do something about it.

D.L.: You feel obligated.

Conrad: Yeah, she always says ''To whom much is given, much is expected.'' I know it's true but you don't hear it in many other families. She used to say it to me a lot because she used to think I was a little bit wayward. I suppose all of this ties into responsibility.

  You know, maybe this isn't related, but you get kind of paranoid about having kids, too.

Kate: I never thought about that.

Conrad: You know, I've always had this longstanding joke about when my wife gets pregnant I'm going to keep her going to the doctor all the time and keep her in the house. It's absolutely the most foolish thing, but in some sense it's kind of serious.

D.L.: You are aware how vulnerable you are.

Kate: I think that's true a lot.

Conrad: And, you even feel guilty about that, you know.

Kate: I don't think I thought so much about having kids. It's more that people can be very strong in the face of adversity like that. That Laura is very strong; it was a very positive thing. They are not strong because it was easy to be strong.

D.L.: They rose to the occasion.

Kate: Yeah. And everyone was very selfless about it. There was an incredible amount of sacrifice, not on our part at all by comparison.

Conrad: Boy, sometimes you speak to Mom and you say, "You must have really sacrificed," and she'll say, "But you did, too." I was just here, you know.

Kate: No, I don't think so. The whole tone of the family was that you had some responsibility to go out and help people.

Conrad: Yes. You definitely do feel a definite responsibility. Some of it's good and some of it's bad. You definitely feel obligated.

Kate (to Conrad): Do you feel like you are not normal?

Conrad: It's hard to know because you don't know how you would have been different. It was like a responsibility immediately from birth. "Go out and help people, son!"

D.L.: That was one of the messages in your family?

Conrad: It was never really said.

Kate: No. It was because they were all doing it. I mean, Poppa was doing it when he was helping with the kids. Everybody was just doing it.

Kate (to Conrad): Do you think you would be different?

Conrad: Oh, yeah, sure.

Kate: How would you be different?

Conrad: I don't know, but I know I would be, but it's [Laura's deafness] just such a part of my identity that I take it for granted. It is so ingrained in me. I know that if I walked out of here and was hit by a car, I would respond differently.

Kate: It's strange that something that has been so much a part of my identity is being reacted to so differently. Now people will talk to you about the deafness and say, "Oh, really. Your sister is deaf." People are really interested and want to know, and they may want to know whether she signs or she speaks. And you get much more of that kind of feedback, whereas before, when you were very young, you would be attacked for it. And it's a very strange thing to be able to say that something that has been part of me is being reacted to in different ways at different times in my life.

D.L.: When you were young, you saw deafness as a stigma?

Kate: Yeah, and you had to be defensive about it. You had to say, "Yeah, but she could still go to school and she could still. . . ."

Conrad: And parents. Don't you think everyone was a bit patronizing to you when you were young because your sister was deaf? Not only kids but parents. They used to react, "Isn't that bad that you are so young and have to deal with this."

And now maybe because I'm grown up, parents say, "Well, that's amazing and how did all that happen?" People, when I was younger, seemed to be more cautious about talking about Laura's deafness. Now, more people want to talk about it.

Kate: Yeah, and now people approach you more respectfully. I think kids, when you are very young, just don't understand. They always felt sorry for me. To defend this, it was hard for me to always say, "Yeah, it is sort of mean and she is my sister and I still love her and we still have a normal family."

D.L.: You also wanted to forget about it and just be plain Kate.

Kate: I think we are just plain Kate and Conrad now. I mean I feel very much now that my Kateness has been nurtured a lot.

Conrad: We are closer because of it.

Kate: I think her deafness definitely did that. I think some of it was that she was away at school.

Conrad: It sounds kind of weird, when we were young I could identify with you [Kate] because Laura was the one who was somehow not normal and you were the one who sort of was.

Kate: When you were younger you used to say that deafness was something that you would "fix" and then Laura was going to be normal. What we have been hearing from her now is that she is no less normal. That deafness is what is normal and what we are saying is that she would not be Laura if she was not deaf. The conversation came up and we asked her what she thought of these cochlea implants and she said, "No way. I'm a deaf person." And we both went, "Oh!" And then we thought about it and said, "We can't imagine you not being deaf either!" Normal is not defined as hearing or not hearing; it is just her. And for her, it is not hearing. It seems very inconsequential when you talk about her now.

Conrad: Yeah. When we were young it was sort of like a sickness. It is just a reality now, and now, as you were saying, it is part of her person.

Kate: That is the way it has always been, only we haven't been able to react to it that way.

D.L.: It sounds like you've stopped seeing her as disabled and now she's just a person who doesn't hear well.

Kate: I think we got a lot of that because of what Mom did. Because, if you were the parent and weren't very aware of what the other kids were feeling and what was going on, then the kids might end up feeling that she was just always a disabled person.

D.L.: So your parents, by respecting your personhood and her personhood, allowed you to all grow.

Kate: Oh, yeah.

D.L.: Did you ever feel responsible for Laura?

Kate: I'm smiling because she is very much more outgoing than either of us. A lot more outgoing and very independent. So her personality makes us think that she is more responsible for us. In a lot of situations, she will just take control.

Conrad: It is very true. Whenever I go out with her, like when we go to a movie, there is a 50 cent discount for deaf people and somehow it would seem if I were deaf, I wouldn't really want to make a scene but she'll go right up to them and say, "Look, I'm deaf and I want my 50 cents."

D.L.: You sort of admire her and it embarrasses you at the same time.

Conrad: That's right. I have real admiration for her.

Kate: Yes, because of her personality, we don't feel very responsible for her.

Conrad: Maybe the responsibility may be not for deafness but for the way she has grown up. She is so protective about her room, and I think maybe because of all the times I used to go into her room that somehow she is a different person than if I had razzed her. But I am a little bit afraid when Laura is deaf because I would not mind going into Kate's room and giving her hell but with Laura being deaf somehow I act differently.

Kate: You feel more sensitive about her?

Conrad: Yeah, which is not as normal for kids growing up. I feel guilty about all those things I did because of her deafness that she reacted to and caused her to become this kind of person.

D.L.: You always felt that you couldn't fight with her the way you could with Kate?

Kate: I always felt I could fight with her, although it was different than fighting with Conrad. She's a good fighter.

Conrad: I didn't feel that at all. I felt more like I had to roll over.

Kate: That could be age.

Conrad: It could be age. She was a lot older.

D.L.: Did she get points for her deafness?

Kate: Well, maybe you did not fight so much with her. Maybe you didn't to the last word. You did not fight more than five minutes.

D.L.: So was it one of the unspoken messages, that Laura was a bit more delicate than anyone else in the family?

Conrad: Gee, it's funny. I think, yes, the message was, "Yes, she is delicate," but the reality was she could give and take as well as any of us. Probably better. Her stuff was more for her. If I saw something of Kate's lying around I might touch it. Laura's stuff seemed to have an aura around it. Like her toothbrush, I would never soap her toothbrush like I might do to Kate.

Kate: It is more that she wouldn't understand that it is just a practical joke. Not so much that we are treating her very differently and isolating her but it's maybe that you think more before you would do it to her. Because she might not understand. Just the way she doesn't understand some idioms or something, out of no fault or no inadequacy. You just have to think about what you are going to do.

Conrad: Yeah. It wasn't because it was Laura's stuff; it was because you had to think that extra second longer because if I had thought that much longer with Kate, I probably wouldn't have soaped her toothbrush either. That's stupid. You tended to think more with Laura.

Kate: That would probably be a good thing to have with everybody you interact with. You could just be a thoughtful person.

D.L.: How did you see your parents' roles in regard to Laura's deafness?

Kate: Certainly it seemed a shared thing. You know the decisions as to where to send her to school always seemed like a shared responsibility. I used to think as to what kind of things my parents did. You know, these deaf committee things and my Mom talked to parent groups, and that was incredible. You knew they never intended to do this. And that's what they do. I wonder if I would be open enough to changes in my life. I really admire them.

Conrad: It always seemed to me that Mom was more knowledgeable about it. Although whenever there was work to be done, Dad would go and do it. You know, when this deaf group needed a guy to lead them, there he was. Sort of pragmatic about the whole thing.

Kate: So you think he did more of the business stuff, and she was more into the people stuff. Yeah, that's true, although I can remember when Laura was at school and they didn't have math, so on Saturday mornings, we sat on the bed and Dad used to teach Laura and me. Every Saturday morning we were there, and that's how I learned how to do math. That was something I wasn't aware of at the time but I bet that is something that most fathers don't do. . . . I think the stereotype is to say that the mother is the one who is more active with the kids but that wasn't always so.

Conrad: I think my mom had more of the day-to-day responsibility but only because she was home more.

D.L.: You also saw them paying back; not only were they giving you the message, but they were demonstrating it in how they lived.

Kate: Yes, I think that is the only reason we believe it. Yeah she could say "accident of birth" as much as she wanted to; unless we could see it, I don't think the message would have sunk in. The harmony of it all is why it worked. Yeah, we have old people among us and we have a deaf sister and we respect everyone. It's not just a group of people living in the same house.

Conrad: Yeah, in dealing with everybody, there was a lot more to keep in mind.

D.L.: You had to keep in mind Laura's deafness and Poppa's age and respect that.

Kate: Yeah, respect.

D.L.: That was another message that you got.

Conrad: I think that they had some more courage having more kids. I think it would be easier for me to have a handicapped kid now. I'm not asking for that now, but it would be easier for us than it was for them. I don't think we can paint the picture as being completely positive, but it is, generally.

Kate: It's that you realize that your expectations are different. You realize you can have a kid and it might not hear. So you say what's really the most important thing? That you have a family where everyone feels good about themselves. Where everyone feels effective. Where everyone feels good about each other. You are brought down to the base level, to what you cannot sacrifice.

D.L.: Laura's deafness kind of helps your get your priorities straight.

Kate: Oh, yes. Oh, definitely. I think it has done that for us. It was a good thing. You know, what can I live without, and what's very important to me; that says more specifically who you are. If you go into the store and you can only get two things, you have to think about what you really need. Laura's deafness just cuts right through. No ambiguity about that.

The Wagner family illustrates many of the notions described in Chapter One. We can certainly see how every member of the family was affected by Laura's deafness. The family as the interconnected system had to survive and grow and accommodate the stresses engendered, not only by the deafness, but by the other life-cycle stresses; such as the death of Lydia's mother, the inclusion of her father into the family, and the births of other children. In all cases, everyone was affected.

It is important to note that a major turning point for Bill and Lydia Wagner came when they realized that Laura was going to "make it." They could then begin to relax; they could hire a tutor; they could lighten up considerably. Up to that point, one gets the feeling that there was a great deal of tension and stress, with everyone focused on Laura's deafness. Professionals need to pay careful attention to the reciprocal nature of parental expectations and the child's performance. When the child starts meeting the expectations, a mutual, positive reinforcement can take place. Where the child fails to meet expectations, often a mutual, negative reinforcement cycle is generated within the parent-child triangular relationship. In this case, the reinforcement was quite positive, and Laura has apparently flourished.

Listening to the Wagners, I think it is possible to deduce some outline of their family paradigm. The family was seen as an important source of strength; in times of crisis, all members pull together. This family has a highly developed sense of responsibility and commitment. Deafness was seen as a family issue and everyone, including Kate and Conrad, had a responsibility to ameliorate the deafness. Implied in this was the notion that Laura was more fragile than anyone else and that her needs predominated in the house. All members of the Wagner family saw deafness as a stigma and they also recognized that they were no longer a normal family.

I think the move to the residential school for the deaf, while based in part on the need to find a suitable program for Laura, also was needed to restore some semblance of normality in the family. The parents were beginning to recognize that the family was being distorted by their total commitment to deafness. The residential placement was an effort, and I think a successful one, to restore homeostasis to the family. Both Bill and Lydia commented on how like a normal family they were when Laura was at school. There was always considerable tension in the household when Laura would return, which again challenged the homeostasis. It had to be very difficult for a family to have to establish a new homeostasis every weekend—to accommodate first Laura's leaving then her return. This put great stress on everyone.

At the present time, the Wagners are on the verge of another paradigmatic shift. They must come to see Laura as an independent adult in the final stages of leaving home; they seem prepared to make this shift.

In many respects, the Wagners fit the model of the optimal family. Their communication seems honest and direct. Their roles were clearly defined and flexible. Lydia clearly had the day-to-day responsibility and Bill was there to fill in when needed. He seemed to be the pointman and would negotiate with outside agencies; he also did lessons when needed. It was clearly a shared responsibility, with Conrad and Kate having their roles, including teaching language to Laura. There was considerable conflict within the familly—the mother-daughter relationship was conflictual and there was fighting among the siblings. Yet, they all liked one another and were able to keep the conflict manageable. This family has been able to maintain stability in the face of much stress and change, and it has utilized well the resources available to it in both its extended family and in the community.

CHAPTER 3

Parents

According to Minuchin (1974), modern parenting is essentially an impossible task. He feels, and I agree wholeheartedly, that "parenting is an extremely difficult task that no one performs to his entire satisfaction, and no one goes through the process unscathed. Probably it was always more or less impossible. In today's complex, fast developing society, in which generational gaps occur at smaller and smaller intervals, parenting difficulties have increased" (p. 83).

There always is conflict within the parental task. Parents cannot protect and guide a child without recourse, at times, to being controling and restrictive. On the other hand, children cannot grow without testing the limits imposed by their parents and thus being seen by their parents as rejecting and hostile. The process of socialization is inherently conflictual, all in the name of love. Parenting requires the capacity to nurture, guide, and control; in order to do this, parents must have executive authority. Parents are not only in conflict with their children, they are also in conflict with themselves as to whether they are fulfilling their nurturing function or their controlling-guiding function. Conflict per se is not bad, although most families try to avoid it. From conflict comes the change in role relationships and expectations necessary to accommodate growth. Children must push against the limits imposed by their parents in order to accommodate the developmental mandate to grow; and parents must grudgingly give ground.

To see the parental function as solely conflictual, I think, is to miss the rewards of the parental process. As I write this sentence, I am reminded of a Somerset Maugham anecdote. The author was feted on the occasion of his 80th birthday. Asked to contribute some closing remarks, he began by saying. "There are many advantages to being 80 years of age." Then, there followed a very long pause, at which the audience became very uncomfortable. "Only I can't think of any," he finally continued, to the relief of everyone. I am not sure I can articulate clearly the parental rewards, as they are often very subtle. There is much joy and growth in parenting, as well as much stress. My children are slowly becoming good friends and good company. We have shared many adventures together. Without begging the issue, parenting is something that one has to experience in order to fully appreciate.

Parenting a deaf child basically is not different from parenting a hearing child. The issues of parenting are fundamentally the same. The deafness, however, imposes an enormous complexity on the process, and each step in parenting requires more thought and more care. I think one of the major mistakes parents of deaf children are most apt to make is to get so caught up in the deafness that they fail to meet the child's developmental and psychological needs-in short, to forget the child underneath the deafness.

Shutz (1971) suggested that there is a hierarchy of human psychological needs beyond the obvious needs for shelter, food, and procreation. He suggested that human beings need affiliation, affection, and control: by affiliation, he means the feeling of belonging; by affection, the feeling of being loved; and by control, the feeling of having power. Affiliation-affection-control is a useful paradigm for looking at the developmental tasks of the child and at the problems of parenting both the hearing child and the deaf child. All children must successfully negotiate these issues in order to achieve satisfaction in living.

HEARING CHILD

Affiliation

The hearing infant's affiliation with the primary caretaker, which is usually the mother, is total. As the child matures, this affiliation constantly broadens. It is the ultimate task of both the parents and the child to differentiate the child from the family, so that he or she can form a new family. The movement is always out of the family. My oldest son gently reminds me when I leave a telephone message for him to call home that he is confused by the message, as he has another home now.

The preschool child identifies with the whole family as opposed to the infant-mother bond. The school-age child begins to establish wider affiliations, by joining groups such as Little League, Scouts, clubs, etc. During adolescence the differentiation process seems to accelerate and the child's peers become the dominant affiliation group. There is very little that I now do that does not acutely embarrass my 17 year old son. When I watch him at his track meets, he might acknowledge my presence by a surreptitious wave of the hand, if he is sure none of his friends is looking. When he was 13, knowing what was coming from my experience with my older son, I took the summer off and spent considerable time with him. At age 14, he would play with me if he could not get a friend; I understood that. After age 15, it was very hard to get him to go any place with me, unless I allowed him to be accompanied by a friend. I know now from my experience with my older son that I will become more acceptable in a few years. I just have to be patient.

A teenager needs to look critically his or her parents and find them wanting. It is part of the final separation process, that each child must undergo. The parents' task is to help the child make that separation. The irony of parenting is that to do the job well is to do oneself out of a job. It is also absolutely essential that parents keep a sense of humor and perspective during this process because at times it is quite painful. My oldest daughter would pick a fight on the eve of any prolonged separation from home. For her, it was always easier to leave mad than sad. Unfortunately, she had to make several passes at it before she could finally separate, which was a bit hard on her parents!

The whole process, though, is very complex. I once heard a psychologist lecture on the "Perfect Parent"—who, recognizing that the adolescent has a great deal of difficulty separating from home, makes life at home uncomfortable for the child. I rushed home from the lecture to tell my wife about it, and she assured me I had nothing to worry about.

Affection

Human beings require affection in order to survive. Infants left in orphanages, cared for physically by attendants, who changed their diapers and fed them but lacked the time to play and coo at the babies, failed to thrive. This disorder, described by Ribble (1943), is known as *marasmus*, from the Greek word meaning "wasting of the body." The solution is simple: Give the infants love and affection and they will grow. This is true all through the parenting process and in all human relations.

Unfortunately, the only time that one sees many parents giving their child unconditional affection is when the child is an infant. The child does not have to do anything but be; he or she is loved just for himself or herself. Affection, because it is so powerful a reinforcing agent, becomes the major means of controling children's behavior. The withdrawal of love, or the threat of it, is used to control children. Parents, and also teachers, send the child so many "I love you if—" messages (I will love you *if* you clean your room, are good, etc.) that the child becomes uncertain if the parents love them for themselves or for their performances. So much self-esteem gets tied up with performance that the child does not always recognize that he or she can be a smart person who sometimes does dumb things or be a good person who sometimes feels and acts hateful. The parents always need to differentiate the child's behavior from the child, so that they dislike what the child does and still like the child; not a very easy thing to do.

It is absolutely fundamental to our self-esteem to recognize that we are loved for ourselves and not for all the good we do. Unfortunately, one sees adults who are never sure that they are loved. These are the fathers who ask "Do they love me for me or my paycheck?" or mothers who wonder whether the child really appreciates them. Such parents usually produce guilt-ridden children with low self-esteem, because they are always seeking reassurance and gratitude from their children.

Control

One of the most cogent issues of parenting is control. It is an issue that occurs throughout the parenting process. Parents must slowly give children control of, and therefore responsibility for, their own lives. The timing of relinquishing control must be very precise. The parents must allow the child enough freedom to explore and grow, at the same time; they must maintain enough control so that the child is not injured. Parents who fail to allow the child enough control send the message that the child is incompetent or that the world is a very dangerous place. Parents who allow the child too much freedom too soon give the child too many negative experiences, and the child may conclude that he or she is incompetent. In either case, one would have a child who avoids risk and has low self-esteem, or one who fails to take responsibility; the parents must tread a very fine line.

The infant has minimal control. Fortunately, the infant seems to have minimal needs. The infant cries and the parent changes a diaper or provides food. If neither works, one finds very frustrated parents and a very frustrated child. The principal means of control of the environment is speech and language. By talking, the child makes his or her wants known and can control the adults; as the child gains more motor ability, he or she can control the physical environment.

As the child grows, the parents must allow more freedom. Invariably, however, there is a lag between the parents' perception of the child's capabilities and the child's own perception, and thus is born conflict between parent and child. I have often thought that "the perfect parent" would have no conflict with his or her children; and that, therefore, I am not a perfect parent. But I am beginning to see that conflict is necessary and desirable. Freedom cannot be given; it must be won. The inevitable conflicts between parents and children teach the children to respond to their own perceptions of reality, to learn to trust themselves and not blindly to trust authority. While, at times, I think how nice it would be to have docile children, I remember the German soldiers who executed all those prisoners because they were so ordered. This thought helps sustain me during conflicts with my children.

The control issue is a constant dilemma for parents. Parents have the wisdom born of having made their own mistakes and want to save their child from making the same errors. It is very painful sometimes to have to allow your own children to make their own mistakes. I have decided that raising children, especially adolescents, becomes almost a religious experience. I have found myself praying a great deal as my children went off to do what I considered dangerous things, which they in their naiveté could not see as dangerous. So I allow my daughter to go on a date with a boy, who looked about 12-years-old and I was sure had just learned to drive. To be a parent of a normal child you have to be very lucky, and, unfortunately for parents of a deaf child, their luck has run out.

THE DEAF CHILD

Affiliation

For the deaf child, affiliation is extremely complex, because over 90 percent of all deaf children have hearing parents. This means that the child can form an affiliation with two possible groups that, at this point in our social consciousness, are fairly disparate. Social issues in deafness have been compared to a minority group dynamic (Rosen, 1986); however, in racial, religious, and ethnic minority groups, the parents also belong to the minority group. This is not the case for the deaf child, and often the family must make a painful choice between the deaf community and the hearing world of the parents.

In a recent parent group with which I was involved, there were two parents who had adopted their children. One mother was fearful that one day her child might seek his biological mother and prefer her over the adoptive mother. The other adoptive mother was very appreciative of the biological mother and wanted to thank her for giving up her son and to assure her that the child was doing well. I think these two parents represent the ambivalence that hearing parents feel towards the deaf community. On the one hand, they are very grateful that the community exists for their child to affiliate with, at the same time, they are fearful that they will lose their child to the deafness. It is the degree to which the parents feel secure in their relationship with their child that they can feel comfortable about the child's access to the deaf community. A parent, or a spouse, who feels secure in the love relationship, does not see outsiders as a threat but as welcome additions to enrich the relationship.

When the child's affiliation needs for the deaf community begin to emerge is very variable and depends in a large part on the parents' attitude towards deafness and the child's school experience. For example, parents who strive so hard to have their child be ''normal'' and feel very threatened by the deaf community usually produce adolescents who at first reject any contact with deaf peers. If these same children, however, cannot establish satisfactory peer relationships with hearing children, they rebel and discover the deaf world. Often these children become very militant deaf adults, who reject the hearing world and their parents. Sometimes, it is not the parents per se who cause the rebellion but a very negative experience that some deaf children undergo at the hands of the hearing world that causes them to very naturally seek comfort and affiliation with the deaf community.

The Wagners tried to bridge the gap between the two worlds. Laura was enrolled in programs predominantly for deaf children until age 11. Her closest friends still are those deaf children she met at the residential school, even though she has been mainstreamed ever since she left that school. The Wagners would like her to have a relationships with a hard-of-hearing boy, not only because of her skill level but, I think, also because, for them, hard of hearing represents a bridge between the deaf and hearing worlds.

The problem of affiliation is an acute one at this stage of our social development because of the militancy of the deaf community, but in some respects, this is a false problem. I do not think any parents, whether they have a hearing child or not, can ever enter their child's world. One of the hardest things a parent has to learn is that he or she can no longer meet all the child's needs. The world is so complex and fast moving that my children's experiences are very different from mine, and I, in many respects, am a stranger to their world. The generational gap is a very real one. We can only share our experiences of family and our loving and caring for one another with our children; all, however, must go their separate ways.

Affection

The affection issue is an acute one for the deaf child because, at the time of diagnosis, parents are invariably upset, and an enormous strain is introduced into the parent-child bond that is not present with parents of a normal child. A mother of a 2-$\frac{1}{2}$ year old deaf child said,

> I am glad I did not tumble to the fact that my child was deaf until she was 14 months old. I really enjoyed her for that first year. I was very carefree in my mothering. When I found out she was deaf, I became stiff and very self-conscious. I was terrified about the hearing aids and I was afraid of making any mistakes. There was no fun or joy then.

This is not an uncommon occurrence. Parents often are devastated by the diagnosis and, for a while, are incapable of giving unconditional regard to the child. Irrational as it may seem, parents are very often angry at their child for being deaf, which can interfere with the father- or mother-infant bond.

Professionals need to be very concerned about the loss of unconditional affection as it relates to the diagnostic process. Too often one finds professional meetings devoted to determining the most efficacious means of identifying an infant as hearing impaired and not often enough, to my mind, on what needs to be done to help the families accept the deaf child. Diagnosis and habilitation need to be discussed simultaneously. I can find no study that demonstrates that very early detection of deafness leads to better functioning deaf adults. I would prefer that diagnosis rapidly follow any parental concern about their child's hearing status rather than professionals imposing their anxiety on the family. Those carefree months of parent-child affection should not be given up lightly, and concommittant with any diagnostic procedure must be intensive habilitation focusing on parental feelings and attitudes.

The relationship between the child's performance and the parents' expectations also affects the parents' ability to give affection. Parents need to see results of their efforts. They need to feel that they can change and affect the course of the handicap; they need to be reinforced by their child. Systems theory tells us that the child has an equal effect on the parents' behavior; there is experimental confirmation as well. Anderson (1981) reviewed several studies of families with a handicapped child and concluded the effect was bidirectional; as the child met or exceeded the parents' expectations, the parents would increase the upper limit of control. In short, they would allow the child more freedom. The converse was also true, that if the child failed to meet parental expectation, the parents imposed further restrictions.

The Wagners found it much easier to relax and enjoy Laura when they began to see her making progress. In some ways, the deaf child carries an awesome burden of his or her parents' self-esteem, and there is a complex interaction between the parents and the child. As the child shows some progress (i.e., meets some parental expectation), the parents can provide more unconditional regard. As the child feels more loved, he or she becomes more responsive, which in turn makes things easier for the parents. The sensitive intercession of the professional early in the habilitation process can affect the nature of the parent-child affection spiral. Parents, for example, need to be able to express their anger and have it accepted. They need also to be convinced of their own power to affect change. This will be discussed in more detail in Chapter Eight.

Control

The area in which parents of hearing-impaired children are most likely to fail in is the assumption of responsibility. It is a difficult area for all parents, but the parents of the deaf child are especially vulnerable in this arena. For one thing, because of unresolved feelings of guilt and feeling of vulnerability, there is a strong tendency for parents to overprotect the child. In addition, there are real areas in which the child cannot perform well. For example, the mother of a 3-year-old deaf child was terrified that her child might get lost and be unable to tell people where he lived. This parent also was afraid to allow the child outside alone with his bicycle, because he might not hear the cars coming. Bill Wagner has constant fears about Laura's naiveté and her lack of "street smarts."

It is always difficult to determine what is a legitimate fear based on an assessment of reality and what is the projection of the parents' guilt and vulnerability. There are many times when parents must "bite the bullet." One is reminded of Lydia Wagner sitting in the car and sending her daughter into the store to shop. It is very painful at times, but also very necessary, for the deaf child to grow by assuming responsibility, which means there are times when the child will fail.

A convincing body of evidence indicates that deaf children and adults are remaining passive and are failing to take responsibility for themselves. Rotter (1966), a social psychologist, developed a test instrument to measure "locus of control." He found that people tended to distribute themselves along a continuum from a an inner locus of control to an external locus of control. Persons who tended to have a greater inner locus of control assumed responsibility for their own behavior and perceptions, were more self-confident in their decisions, and were less likely to seek authority for guidance. Indivduals with an external locus of control tended to blame events forces outside themselves, were less confident in making decisions, and often saw themselves as powerless. Individuals with an external locus of control seldom took responsibility for their own behavior. Bodner and Johns (1977) administered the Rotter scale to 38 high-reading deaf students and their hearing controls. (They had to use high-reading students because the test vocabulary proved too complex for the majority of the deaf students originally selected.) They found that the deaf students were significantly more external in their locus of control than the hearing students. Dowaliby, Burke, and McKee (1983) constructed a paper and pencil research instrument that measured internality, externality, and people orientation. They administered the test to 267 students entering the National Training Institute for the Deaf and to a control sample of 100 normally hearing undergraduates. Results indicated that the hearing-impaired students were substantially more external in their locus of control than the hearing students.

White (1982) reported on a series of workshops he conducted with teachers and counselors at six schools for the deaf. He asked the 281 participants to rank in order of need 24 social competencies that the students needed to develop. Failure to accept responsibility for one's actions ranked as the number one need and, therefore, the number one priority for amelioration. Brice (1985), found that deaf first- and fourth-grade children were much more tolerant of ambiguity than the control group of hearing children. The children were shown series of animal pictures that gradually became distorted. For example, the child was shown a rabbit that, as more cards were turned, slowly became a turtle. The child had to name the animal on each card. Scores were based on how long it took a child to notice the distortion and to ask for an explanation for the change. The results of the study showed that the hearing children were significantly quicker than the deaf ones to respond to the changes in the pictures and to demand an explanation. The deaf children remained more passive and were less inclined to question and explore their cognitive and social world than the hearing children.

Loeb and Sarigiani (1986) compared the self-perceptions of mainstreamed hearing-impaired children with mainstreamed visually impaired children and with children who have no major sensory impairments. They found that the hearing-impaired children had a more external locus of control and lower self-confidence than either of the other groups.

The roots of the external locus of control of deaf children may lie in the child-rearing practices of their parents. Cook (1963), analyzing the child-rearing attitudes of mothers of deaf children, found that they tended to be overprotective and overindulgent. Freeman, Malkin, and Hastings (1975) compared the interview results of 120 families with a deaf child and a control sample of families with a hearing child and found that the mothers of deaf children permit them to do significantly less than do mothers of hearing children; the difference was somewhat less marked for fathers. Wedell-Monnig and Lumley (1980) observed matched pairs of mothers of young deaf children with mothers of hearing children and found that the deaf children were more passive and less actively involved in interaction than their hearing counterparts. The mothers of deaf children were always more dominant in their interaction with their children than mothers of hearing children. The authors attribute this behavior in part to the deaf children's "learned helplessness."

I think it is clear from the research evidence that current populations of deaf students tend to be passive, with an externally oriented locus of control and a lower self-esteem. I am not sure who is to blame for this. I suspect it may be due in part to an unconscious conspiracy of both teachers and parents to overprotect the deaf child, so as to save him or her from further harm or mistakes; in the process they have been limiting the child's passage into adulthood.

PARENTAL FEELINGS

Probably the model most frequently used to explain the parental process of acceptance of their child's hearing impairment has been the grief reaction, stemming from the pioneering work of Kubler-Ross (1969) in her observations of terminally ill patients. Her model of the grief process includes (1) denial, (2) anger, (3) bargaining, (4) depression, and (5) acceptance. Tanner (1980) wrote a comprehensive article on the grief reaction and how this relates to the speech pathologist and audiologist. Drotar, Baskiewicz, Irvin, Kennell, and Klaus (1975) studied parental reactions to their children who had congenital malformations. Based on intensive interviews, they were able to note five stages of parental reaction: shock, denial, sadness and anger, adaptation, and reorganization. I have used the Kubler-Ross model of adaptation in my previous writings (Luterman, 1979). I think it is a generally useful way of describing parental reactions. I have, however, grown wary of it; it presents a simplistic view of a very complex process and, as such, can be misleading. Almost all models of the grief process imply an orderliness that is not there; the stages of grief are not mutually exclusive and there are no clear demarcation between one stage and another. Acceptance itself is not devoid of grief, as is implied in the model; it is characterized by a sadness that no longer is immobilizing. The father of a 15 year old described it as, ''At first you hurt like hell and then it becomes a dull ache that does not go away.''

Coming to grips with a terrible loss is a fluid process and I find it useful to describe the various feelings that parents may have and then to examine the implications of these feelings on parental behavior. The expression of these feelings will vary widely from family to family.

Shock, Anxiety

Shock is the initial reaction to the diagnosis of deafness, or more aptly, to the realization that the hearing loss is permanent. The shock reaction is a self-protective mechanism, much like denial, that is an emotional divorce from the proceedings. One mother described it as ''seeing herself on a stage and going through the motions, commenting 'This is very interesting.' '' At this point, parents can still act and usually show prodigious amount of energy (e.g., traveling to several doctors and having an infinite array of audiological examinations); however, the cognitive and emotional aspects of their being are unhooked from each other: they cannot process much information; they are not psychologically in control of the situation; they feel as if they are hollow shells or automatons going through the motions. They are attempting to keep at bay the very powerful feelings of overwhelming anxiety and fear.

All parents, whether or not they have a handicapped child, at times feel inadequate in the face of the awesome tasks of raising a young child to responsible adulthood. When parents learn that they have a child with special needs, it means that they are going to be challenged to be a "special" parents. This provokes a great deal of fear. Parents never have to be reminded of their responsibility; they know it full well. The feelings of inadequacy lead the parent to seek a savior, someone to rescue them from their own inadequacies. As one father aptly put it, "I am looking to find a quarterback for my family." (He actually wanted a quarterback who would not make any mistakes!) Professionals who work with parents all too often see themselves as the rescue agent and are all too willing to call the "plays"—although doing so convinces the parents that they really are inadequate, that they need someone to call the plays. The only role I accept for such a family, and all families, is as an enthusiastic fan, convinced of the parents' own competency to call a good "game," although not necessarily error free.

Anger, Depression

Almost all parents of hearing-impaired children are quite angry at some fundamental level. Anger comes from a violation of expectations. Parents have many expectations about their unborn children, not the least of which is that they will be normal. When they find that the child does not hear normally and cannot be cured, they feel cheated and wonder why they were singled out. Anger also comes about when there is a loss of control: When we can no longer operate in our own best interests. Having a handicapped child means losing degrees of personal freedom. The parent who cannot accept a promotion in his or her company if to do so would mean moving to a community that had no programs for deaf children is angry. The family that does move in order for the child to go to a school for the deaf, and consequently gives up much in their home community, is also very angry.

There is another anger, almost rage, that comes from the frustration of not being able to help their children. All parents I have met, at some level, not always apparent to professionals, want to do right by their children; want to make things better. I can remember so vividly going to the hosital to visit my daughter, who had broken her leg in a car accident and was in a great deal of pain. There was nothing I could do to ease her pain. I felt so angry and frustrated that I wanted to smash something. This is the anger in which one kicks the cat or puts a fist through a door; anybody who crosses my path had better watch out. This type of anger is very often born of frustration and is frequently displaced onto others.

I have found that most people and families do not have good means for expressing anger. Anger is a very threatening emotion. When it is expressed, it is generally equated with loss of love. In actuality, there is a great deal of caring in anger; it implies that the person is very much affected by the situation because the other person means so much. The opposite of love is not anger but indifference. Many families do not allow a direct expression of anger, and thus it is frequently repressed; and such repression can lead to depression. In depression, people often appear devoid of energy and feeling; actually, the feelings are so intense that an immense battle is taking place within the person. The anger is seeking to emerge and the person, not necessarily consciously, is trying to suppress the rage. This leaves little energy to do anything else. It is also true that when we choose to suppress any feeling, we tend to suppress all feelings, and the world becomes a rather gray place.

I think most professionals intuitively recognize that parents are potential emotional volcanos, which might erupt at any time. Very often the anger the parents feel toward their situation is displaced onto the professional. I think most professionals are more afraid of the anger emerging than they are of the grief. Anger is a useful emotion. There is a great deal of energy in anger that needs to be released and directed into programs that benefit all hearing-impaired children. The anger that is turned inward and becomes depression is not used in the best interests of the child. It festers and drains the parents of any useful energy. Professionals need to be prepared to have parents, at some time in their relationship, be angry with them. This is very hard to do.

Guilt, Resentment

Almost all mothers of deaf children feel, at some level, that they are responsible for their child's deafness. Guilt, in general, seems to be epidemic among women in our society. They pick up guilt like a magnet attracts iron filings. I think this stems from our child-rearing practices, which tend to use guilt as a means of controling girls' behavior. One mother in a group said once, "I even feel guilty when it rains." When it comes to bearing a deaf or disabled child, the opportunities for feeling guilty are manifold, since almost 50 percent of the time the cause of the deafness is not known. Parental search for the cause frequently stems from their guilt feelings and represents a desire to fix blame somewhere else. This is not to imply that the search is always a reflection of guilt: parents are also quite legitimately concerned about cause in determining whether or not to have more children.

According to Myerson (1983), "the inevitable guilt that parents of handicapped children experience is really self-directed anger, a feeling or even a conviction that if they had done something differently their child would have been all right" (p. 287). Almost all mothers of congenitally deaf children, in which there is no known etiology, have a guilty secret. It is almost impossible to have a nine-month pregnancy without something untoward happening that, when one looks in retrospect, could be blamed for the deafness. Thus, one mother felt she caused the deafness because she failed to take her vitamin pills; another, because she wore high heels and fell down; a third, because she went to a party and had several drinks. Although most of these guilty secrets are unfounded and cannot withstand rational examination, they often lead to unwholesome behavior.

Fathers, too, are frequently guilt-ridden. This guilt, however, stems from a failure to fulfill their perceived role in the family. Most father/husbands are assigned, or assign themselves, the role of family protector. It is their job to make things better for everyone. When they cannot take away the pain of their wife or the pain experienced by their handicapped child, they feel guilty.

Sondra Diamond (1981), a remarkable person with severe cerebral palsy, described her father's guilt as "It is not guilt over having done something wrong by bearing or siring a disabled child, but, rather, guilt in terms of not having done the best for the child. He used examples such as feeling he could have explored other possible therapy treatments and feeling he could have smoothed more of the hurt that I was exposed to as a result of being disabled."

Guilty parents are driven parents, almost always seeking the cause when it is no longer relevant and their energy could be better spent in child management activities. Guilt-driven parents tend to overprotect their child. They feel "I let something bad happen to you once and I'm not going to let it happen again." They do not let their child have the normal experience necessary to develop the skills needed for responsible adulthood, which include taking risks and getting some "bloody noses," occasionally.

Guilty parents also are not very trusting of professional competency, questioning teachers and audiologists frequently and seeking other opinions, when neither seem at all justified by the situation. It is very hard to maintain a long-term relationship with a guilt-driven parent.

The flip side of feeling guilty is feeling resentment. Guilt is such an uncomfortable feeling that we also resent the person or thing that is "making" us feel guilty. Guilt, when used as a controling device in a relationship, as occurs in many families, usually leads to unhappy, poorly functioning families. The resentment simmers and generally sabotages relationships. Guilt-driven people usually "forget" to do important things, frequently miss appointments, and become unreliable. Resentments tend to lead toward passive-aggressive behavior rather than anger, which can lead to direct action where more energy is available for making changes.

Vulnerability, Overprotection

For many parents, having a deaf child is the first bad thing that has happened to them. Very frequently, this leaves them stunned and bewildered. If you live long enough, something bad will happen to you; and if you don't live long enough, something bad already has happened to you. This is one of the facts of our existence. We tend to protect ourselves from the anxiety this engenders by thinking ourselves invulnerable. Since we are all at risk, our fantasy of being invulnerable is also at risk and when the bad thing does happen, it increases anxiety. Lydia Wagner moved out of the house when her husband developed cold sores during her second pregnancy, and both Conrad and Kate are much more aware of the potentiality of handicaps in their children and in their own lives.

The parents also begin to think "Something bad has happened to my child once, and I'm not going to let any other bad thing happen again." For example, a mother whose normally hearing child was deafened by meningitis said,

> When I got her home from the hospital, I wouldn't let her out of the yard to play with any other children. I was terrified if anyone even coughed near her. I didn't let her ride in the cart at the supermarket because I am afraid of germs. I sometimes took a can of disinfectant and sprayed the cart before I put her in it. Last week, she had a fever and I cried for several hours, sure she was going to have meningitis again or her hearing was going to get worse. . . . I am so scared.

Vulnerable parents respond very much like guilty parents and tend to overprotect their children with, as the research evidence shows, bad consequences for the children.

Confusion, Panic

Confusion is a normal stage early in the learning process when we attempt to acquire any new information. The vocabulary itself is so unfamiliar that we are often stuck trying to recall what a given word or term means and lose the meaning of the sentence itself. Terms such as *frequency, decibel,* and *audiogram* are unfamiliar to most persons. Yet, professionals, who almost literally live with these terms, use them quite freely with parents, perhaps defining them once and then assuming that the parents understand; they forget that it takes patience and time. Professionals also frequently forget that parents are approaching the learning process with a high degree of anxiety, which limits their cognitive ability. In my experience, parental confusion and panic is not caused by too little information. The parents have been given too much too soon. Not only are they supplied information by professionals, but they are also getting advice from well-meaning relatives, friends, and even strangers, who notice their child's hearing aids and feel obligated to tell about their own experiences. To have a deaf child means to lose one's anonymity; strangers often give themselves permission to approach the parents and offer unsolicited advice or encouragement.

Parents feel very often as though they are drowning in a sea of information, much of it conflicting. This leads to panic, which can be immobilizing; parents who cannot seem to make a decision are frequently immobilized by their panic.

Denial

Probably no single reaction within the grief process is so misunderstood or confounds the parent-professional relationship more than denial. Denial must be seen as a very normal psychological reaction to a situation that is perceived as being overwhelming. It is self-protective and occurs spontaneously and unconsciously; it is designed to ward off excessive anxiety. Thus, when I am driving my car and it begins to make strange noises, I respond by turning on the radio. On the surface, this is very strange behavior. I know that turning on the radio is not going to solve my crisis but it makes me feel better in the face of a potential catastrophe. Because I can no longer hear the noises, the noises no longer exist for me.

No matter how well-prepared the parents may be for the diagnosis of deafness, there will be some elements of denial in their response and their behavior. When the professional does not understand this denial, it looks as if the parents are derelict in their duty and are hurting the child by not following through on the recommended clinical management. Denial extends to anything that will objectify the deafness, e.g., hearing aids, use of sign language, or any association with other parents of deaf children. Parents who are reluctant to put a hearing aid on a child or to attend a signing class or a group session for parents of deaf children can be, and are, almost invariably seen by audiologists and educators as "bad" parents, who are hurting the child. These parents are in denial.

Invariably, the professional's anger at the parents emerges in admonitions, telling the parents how important it is to keep the hearing aid on the child, to attend classes, etc. These lectures only increase the distance between the parents and the professional and do nothing to help the parents give up the denial reaction. The parents will almost invariably agree verbally with the audiologist—they know the hearing aid is important—then, for some reason, forget to put the hearing aid on the child. Thus begins an unwholesome cycle, with the parents looking more and more like bad parents, while trying to hide their behavior in the face of an angry, admonishing audiologist. This unhealthy relationship leads to both a frustrated audiologist and frustrated parents. Invariably, in such situations, there is a mutual "turn-off" and, unfortunately, it is not uncommon to see parents of adolescents who have never been allowed to work through the denial process and have very impaired relationships with all professionals. Tragically, they almost invariably have poorly functioning children.

Denial must be seen as a function of feeling overwhelmed: It is a plea for help; a crisis of confidence. If I felt confident in my ability to fix engines, then psychologically I could afford to "hear" the engine knocking. I would pull the car over to the side of the road and set about repairing it. In short, I would operate in a rational and approved manner; however, as long as I felt inadequate, I needed to protect myself by denying the problem. This is a normal reaction. Lectures that attack my behavior are not helpful; in fact, they just serve to increase my feelings of inadequacy. What I need, and what all parents need, is someone to listen sensitively to my fear and to help me gain confidence in my own ability to solve my problems: When that happens I can give up denial.

THE REACTION TO CRISIS

The parents' reactions to the deafness of their children are very complex and unique to each family, depending in large part on the parents' previous experiences and expectations. For some, very often middle-class parents, the child's deafness is the first bad thing that has happened to them. They are devastated, sometimes responding almost with indignation that such a thing should happen to them. For other parents, often lower-class parents, the deaf child is only one more bad thing in a series of bad things that are happening to them. They will often respond with a shrug and a sigh of resignation. A family crisis depends on the degree to which the family members regard an event as changing their lives in an undesirable manner. The deaf child introduces the potentiality of a crisis, rather than being the actual crisis: The crisis is not in the event but in the response to the event. I have met parents with a deep religious sense, for example, who do not seem to be devastated by their child's deafness. They seem to calmly accept the child and their mission in life as God's will. Then, they systematically go about the task of habilitating their child. These parents seem to need a minimum of professional intervention. Each family must be approached individually, with the professional listening carefully to the family members.

Parents frequently try to assuage their pain by thinking that the deafness is not so bad, i.e., that there are so many worse disorders. I don't think that this is an effective strategy, as it leaves the parents feeling guilty when they do grieve. With this point of view, they don't give themselves the right to feel pain. Parents must come to acknowledge that it does hurt to have a deaf child, and they must give themselves permission to occasionally experience the grief; then they can get on with the process of habilitating the child. The unacknowledged grief leads to long term pain and is frequently debilitating.

MacKeith (1973) found that there are four major crisis areas for parents:

1. When the parents learn that their child is handicapped.
2. When the child begins receiving services.
3. When the child leaves home and school. (This is the crisis that the Wagners currently are facing, with Laura's impending graduation from college.)
4. When the aging parents can no longer care for their child.

I think these are useful guidelines for recognition of crises, but by no means are they the only ones. Any change can initiate a crisis reaction by the parents, although the change may look relatively minor to an outsider, such as moving a child from a mainstreaming program to a day class program. Crisis is always in the eye of the beholder. The Wagners were able to make numerous changes with seeming ease, as the need for change was apparent and they explored their options carefully. I think the key to successfully making changes and meeting crises is self-confidence, and the Wagners had a full measure of it.

Experiments confirm the value of parental, especially maternal, self-confidence. Gallagher, Cross, and Scharfman (1981) identified the characteristics of parents who were judged by professionals to have made a successful adjustment to the birth of a handicapped child. The data suggested that the major sources of strength were the personal qualities of the parents, and the quality of the husband and wife relationship. Two personal characteristics were associated highly with success. Maternal ego strength and self-confidence and a commitment to a set of supporting values; e.g., religion. The fathers and mothers in the successful families were satisfied with the roles carried by each in the family, whereas in less successful families role satisfaction was lower.

Venters (1981) interviewed 100 families in which there was a child with cystic fibrosis. The families were divided into those who were successful or not successful in coping. She found that families who coped best with the child's disease were those families in which there was a sharing of the burden, both within and outside the family. Successful families also were able to find philosophic meaning in their child's illness, which enabled them to remain optimistic and self-confident in coping with the progress of the disease.

EFFECTS OF DEAFNESS ON MARRIAGE

Marriages are not made in heaven, they are made by imperfect human beings on earth. A successful marriage requires constant work and a smooth blending of the personal paradigms to form the family paradigm. There has to be both similarity of values and comfort and agreement with the role allocation. The introduction of a deaf child will produce stress in the marriage, as both Lydia and Bill Wagner attested. Their roles were clear: Lydia had the principal responsibility for child-rearing, while Bill was the back-up and support person. But their roles were not rigid; he filled in and relieved Lydia of many of the tutorial functions. He also was the point man on making the changes. While Lydia did the research, Bill talked to the educators. Both parents believe strongly in service to others and were active in promoting programs for deaf children and helping other families. Laura's deafness became a centralizing focus for their marriage, and most of their social contact was with other parents of deaf children. While Laura's deafness brought stress, it also seemed to strengthen the marriage bond.

The effects of a handicapped child on a marriage are equivocal. For example, Gath (1977) studied 30 families with a Down's syndrome child for five years after the birth of the child, as well as a carefully controlled group of 30 families with a normal child. At the end of the five year period she found that 9 of the families with a Down's syndrome child experienced severe marital discord. None of the control families reported any severe difficulties. On the other hand, Kazak and Marvin (1984) found that, in 56 families in which there was a child with spinal bifida, a significant portion of parents in the study reported their marriage was strengthened as a result of the handicapped child.

Research on the effects of a deaf child on the parental marriage is not very clear cut. Freeman et al. (1975) found that the incidence of divorce and separation were no greater in families with a deaf child than in the matched control families in the Vancouver area. In a study of 100 English families with a deaf child, Gregory (1976), with true English restraint, tried to assess the impact of the deaf child on the marriage. She found that 23 percent of the parents felt closer as a result of the deafness of their child, while 24 percent felt it was a strain, 25 percent of the families felt that it varied, and 28 percent felt there was no difference.

This spread of responses generally agrees with my clinical impression that the deafness of the child can operate in many different ways on a marriage, at times strengthening the bond and, at different times and in different families, being a very divisive event. I do not think that the deaf child's presence causes divorces per se, but it adds stress on what already may be a potentially weak relationship. For example, the divorced mother of a child deaf due to meningitis said,

> I first realized how weak my husband was when my daughter got meningitis and he just fell apart. I was the one who had to talk to the doctors and make all the decisions. He just divorced himself from the whole thing, and eventually from me.

On the other hand, a mother of a 5 year old said,

> I really grew to appreciate my husband these last few years. He has really risen to the occasion. He has gone with me to all important meetings and he takes over a great deal of the day-to-day responsibility from me. I never knew he cared so deeply for me and my child until this happened.

According to Tavormina, et al. in an unpublished study, as reported by Gallagher et al. (1981), there are four major styles of adapting to the crisis of having a handicapped child. In the first style, the father emotionally divorces himself from the child, leaving the care of the child entirely to the mother, while he involves himself in other outside activity. In the second style, both parents reject the child, which usually results in institutionalization. The third scenario occurs when the parents make the child the center of their universe and subordinate everything else in the family to the service of the handicapped child. The fourth style is identified by the parents' mutual support of the child and each other, while maintaining a sense of their own identity and a semblance of a normal family life.

The fourth style appears to be the one of the optimal family; and in many ways, the Wagners fit that style. I think they sensed that they were becoming a deafness-dominated family, however, and they institutionalized their daughter in order to provide her with a maximal educational experience as well as to maintain a normal family life. Institutionalization per se does not mean rejection. It sometimes is the best solution to a very difficult situation.

Future Children

A hidden effect of deafness on the family is the decision to have future children. The decision to have more children is always difficult for parents to make. The decision rests in large part on their perception of the degree to which deafness handicaps the child and their confidence in their ability to manage the stress caused by the deafness. Economic and religious considerations enter into the picture, too. The sibling position also is critical. If the deaf child is the first child in the familly, many parents will want to risk having another because, as Bill Wagner noted, he wanted to prove that he could have a "normal" child. If the deaf child is a younger child in the family, then very often the parents stop having more children. Sometimes, parents think that having had one handicapped child grants them immunity from having anything else bad happen to them. Unfortunately, life does not work out that way, and parents have gone on to have a second and even a third deaf child.

Parental Needs

Parents who adopt the third coping style, complete dedication to their child, to the exclusion of everything else, frequently have enormous difficulties letting go of their child, as all effective parents must eventually do. These parents' lives very often revolve around deafness and they do not develop other aspects of themselves. "Losing" their child means losing their roles and commitments in life. This is so threatening that they fight to keep the child dependent on them. A mother of an 18 year old said,

> When he left to go to Gallaudet I wanted to pack my bags and go with him. I felt lost. For the first time in a long time I had no P.T.A. meetings, no teachers to meet, and no medical or audiological examination to go to. I felt partly scared, and partly free, also. It was very strange.

The Wagners are at that point where they must let go and, despite Bill's concern about Laura's ability to get a job, he also trusts her to do it. He has not provided her a job in his business, which would be an easy solution. Bill and Lydia, as in all maturing marriages, are now directing their energy from parental issues to marital issues.

Effective clinical management by professionals must help the parents maintain a healthy balance between meeting the needs of the deaf child and meeting their own needs as well. At first, this seems paradoxical because professionals tend to see the deafness as the overriding issue, but we must take a broader view. I think we are working in the child's best interest when we can convince the parents to take some time off for themselves. If there is one thing I have learned over the past 20 odd years of working with parents, it is that happy, fulfilled parents turn out better deaf children than unhappy ones.

REFERENCES

Anderson, C. (1981). The handicapped child's effects on parent-child relations: A useful model for school psychologists. *Psychologists, 10* (1), 82–90.

Bodner, B. & Johns, J. (1977). Personality and hearing impairment: A study in locus of control. *Volta Review, 79,* 362–368.

Brice, P. A. (1985). A comparison of levels of tolerance for ambiguity in deaf and hearing school children. *American Annals of the Deaf, 130* (3), 226–230.

Cook, J. J. (1963). Dimensional analysis of childrearing attitudes of parents of handicapped children. *American Journal of Mental Deficiency, 68,* 354–361.

Diamond, S. (1981). Growing up with parents of a handicapped child: A handicapped person's perspective. In J. L. Paul (Ed.), *Understanding and working with parents of children with special needs.* New York: Holt, Rinehart and Winston.

Dowaliby, F., Burke, N., & McKee, B. (1983). A comparison of hearing impaired and normally hearing students on locus of control, people orientation, and study habits and attitudes. *American Annals of the Deaf*, *128*, 53–59.

Drotar, D., Baskiewicz, A., Irvin, N., Kennell, J., & Klaus, M. (1975). The adaptation of parents to the birth of an infant with a congenital malformation: A hypothetical model. *Pediatrics*, *56* (5), 710–716.

Freeman, R., Malkin, S. & Hastings, S., (1975). Psychosocial problems of deaf children and their families: A comparative study. *American Annals of the Deaf*, *120*, 391–405.

Gallagher, J. J., Cross, A., & Scharfman, W. (1981). Parental adaptation to a young handicapped child: The father's role. *Journal of the Division for Early Childhood*, *3*, 3–14.

Gath, A. (1977). The impact of an abnormal child upon the parents. *British Society of Psychiatry*, *130*, 405–410.

Gregory, S. (1976). *The deaf child and his family*. New York: John Wiley and Sons.

Kubler-Ross, E. (1969). *On death and dying*. New York: Macmillan.

Kazak, A. & Marvin, R. (1984). Differences, difficulties and adaptations: Stress and social networks in families with a handicapped child. *Family Relationships*, *33*, 67–77.

Loeb, R., & Sarigani, P. (1986). The impact of hearing impairment on the self perceptions of children. *Volta Review*, *88*, 89–99.

Luterman, D. (1979). *Counseling parents of hearing impaired children*. Boston: Little, Brown and Co.

MacKeith, R. (1973). The feelings and behavior of parents of handicapped children. *Developmental Medicine and Child Neurology*, *15*, 524–527.

Minuchin, S. (1974). *Families and family therapy*. Cambridge, MA: Harvard University Press.

Myerson, R. (1983). Family and group therapy. In M. Seligman (Ed.), *The family with a handicapped child: Understanding and treatment*. Orlando, FL: Grune and Stratton Inc.

Ribble, M. A. (1943). *The rights of infants*. New York: Columbia University Press.

Rosen, R. (1986). Deafness: A social perspective. In David Luterman (Ed.), *Deafness in perspective*. San Diego, CA: College-Hill Press.

Rotter, J. B. (1966). *Generalized expectancies for internal versus external control of reinforcement*. *Psychological Monographs*, *80* (1, whole No. 609).

Shutz, W. C. (1971). *HERE COMES EVERYBODY*. New York: Harper and Row.

Tanner, D. C. (1980). Loss and grief: Implications for the speech language pathologists and audiologists. *ASHA 22*, 916–921.

Venters, M. (1981). Familial coping with chronic and severe childhood illness: The case of cystic fibrosis. *Social Science and Medicine*, *15A*, 289–297.

Wedell-Monnig, F., & Lumley, J. (1980). Child deafness and mother child interaction. *Child Development*, *51*, 766–774.

White, K. (1982). Defining and prioritizing the personal and social competence needed by hearing impaired students. *Volta Review*, *84*, 266–271.

CHAPTER 4

Family in Practice:
The Murphys

There are seven members of the Murphy family. The parents, Paul and Jean, are high school graduates. Jean has always been a housewife; Paul works for the telephone company. There are five children: the oldest, Sara (26) lives in Hawaii and is a speech therapist working with deaf children; Lynda (24) is working as a receptionist in California; Michael (23), who lives with his parents, is currently teaching in a special education program; Robert (22), the deaf child, works as a dormitory counselor at a school for the deaf in the vicinity, coming home on weekends. He is a graduate of that school. The youngest child is Nicole (10), who has Down's syndrome. Michael was present during the interview.

D.L.: Can you tell me about your experience with Robert?

Jean: In my fifth month of pregnancy, I got German measles. I was told by my pediatrician not to worry, because it would only affect the child during the first three months. So I did put it out of my mind. So we just felt he was fine when he was born. But I had three other kids who were close in age; it was very easy to notice that he wasn't turning and responding to all the noise. So we began to suspect something was wrong at about 6 weeks of age. We first brought him to the pediatrician when he was about 2 months old. The pediatrician sent us to the ear specialist, who sent us to the hospital, because he didn't have equipment to test him. When we got to the hospital, he was about 4 months old, with all this going on and us feeling panicky. By that point, we were just waiting for the doctor to tell us he was deaf. We wanted to hear it because there was so much tension just trying to figure out what was wrong. And they told us he was profoundly deaf. And we started him right away in therapy at the hospital, and then we went to several different nurseries. I was taking him two or three times a week. It was just one-on-one therapy. And then we went to Emerson when he was about 18 months old. And we had a lot of problems with him—eating problems. He wouldn't chew cookies or crackers. He would gag. They told us he was malnourished. A psychologist told us that he was retarded. He was just a very slow child. I think all of that was because he was the fourth child, and when he was born, Sara was 4 and Lynda was 2, and I had Michael in between so I had him in the playpen a lot, and I think his development was slow. I tried to explain that when I went for these tests. It really did a job on me listening to people saying, "Well, what are you doing to him?" I knew I was doing the best I could with all the children concerned, and also taking Robert to those therapies. I didn't think there was a lot of understanding on their part about all my other problems. We went through a lot of traumatic things. He didn't walk until he was 3 because he was in the playpen all the time. Emerson was the godsend of our life.

Paul: Yes.

Jean: I wish there was something like this for the retarded because the idea of the parents having the attention being put on them and their problems was very important. It set the pace not only for Robert but for Nicole, because I've used so many things I learned from that, and we really enjoyed these two years we were involved with Emerson. One of the nicest things you did was one time when we came in with our other children—I don't know if Michael remembers it—and we went and spent the morning in Boston with our other children. It really gave them some attention because they had to go through a lot, too.

After that, he went to a day class for two years. When he was 5, we moved him to another day class, and that is the school that Nicole is now going to; and the same principal, believe it or not, is giving us a hard time now. He stayed there until all the teachers were telling us we had to get him into some other program. So we checked out all the schools for the deaf, and since we didn't want him to live at school, we sent him to one close to home. He went to the school for the deaf as a day student for about five years, and then he went to an integrated junior high school program and then high school. After that, he tried to go to Gallaudet for one year and he did terribly. They told him that he had to take more courses at home to show them that he was really interested in school before he could come back. So, then he went to U. Mass. and did real good there. He didn't have a full course load and he could handle it. And he was very active in the Theater of the Deaf in Boston. But he really wanted to be in the deaf world. He wanted to go back to Gallaudet desperately. He just didn't want to be in the hearing world. So he went back to Gallaudet, got involved with football, and that's about it. When he got back, there was no scholastic work and they told him again he was not ready. He came out and he got a job in a computer assembly plant. And then he got the job at the school for the deaf. He keeps saying he wants to go back to school but he still doesn't have any idea what he wants to do. He's 22 but very immature. His social life is still the most important thing to him right now.

D.L.: Paul, where were you in all this?

Paul: I was working hard. There were times during the 1960s when I worked a lot of overtime and I wasn't home a lot of times when I might have been home.

D.L.: You felt guilty about it?

Paul: Yes, I did. She had all the burdens at the time. But, at the time, it was a matter of economics. I think you had to work overtime in order to make ends meet. Now, I am home other than normal working hours; the overtime is not there.

Jean: But it gave us a good life and it gave me the chance to stay home.

Paul: That overtime was a must at that time.

D.L.: What did you see as your role with Robert?

Paul: I didn't have that much to do with Robert. Jean had all the responsibilities. She had to take him different places and she had to go because I was working. I don't think there was anything else I could have done at the time.

Jean: Well, you always came to the evening meetings.

Paul: I did go to most meetings. I was able to help her in that way. I made time to go to meetings. It was the best thing I could do at the time.

D.L.: So Jean had all the major responsibility?

Paul: She had *all* the major responsibility. She has it right now with

Nicole, too. When there were decisions to change programs, we always talked them over and we always sat down and made decisions together. Most of the times it was Jean's decisions and I probably went along with it more or less because she knew most things that were going on.

Jean: I think it was more or less like that because I would do all the talking and visiting and I'd come home and tell him all about it. I hated it. I wanted him to help make the decisions; I wish he could have visited with me. If I make the mistake, it's always going to be my fault. Although he's never done that. He's never said, ''we shouldn't have done that.''

Paul: It's the same thing now with Nicole. She makes the decisions because I don't see the things she does.

Jean: Lots of times when I have to go to these educational planning meetings, I get traumatized. It's coming up again and I'm scared. I would like him to go and me stay home, but that is not always possible. I'm worried that he would go and not do everything I want. So I have to go.

D.L.: When did Robert begin to sign?

Jean: That's an interesting thing. When he was at the school for the deaf, total communication began to come in and they started in the lower grades. He was in the upper class and they did not sign there, and Robert hated signs. When he went to the junior high school and they had to have the signs (they did it with the interpreter going to the classes and all), Robert fought against it. We had more trouble with him about those signs. He fought going to the classes. He didn't want to have anything to do with it. His friends were hearing. Then, we really don't know what happened to him when he got to high school; it was like a complete turnaround. It was like he didn't want us. He didn't want anybody but his deaf friends and it's more or less stayed that way. A lot of the teachers were teaching about deaf culture and about deaf power. I really resented a lot of it because I felt that they were turning him to the other side without any encouragement to be with hearing people at all. Then, I noticed all of a sudden that he wasn't going to speech therapy classes and they weren't pushing it. It meant everything was going down the drain, all the years we worked so hard for everything. There was no fighting him about it.

We went through so much turmoil. We kept thinking "Did we do the right thing?" He was changing so. The three years he was in high school were very hard.

D.L.: It was almost like a rejection of you.

Jean: Yeah. It was really. But I think it was the feeling that he rejected everything that we did. He objected to everything we had done previously. You know, all that running around I did. Did I make a big mistake? And then on the other hand, I was worried did he make a big mistake, and I couldn't do anything at that point to sway him.

D.L. (to Michael): How did all this look to you?

Michael: I was so close to him in age that I got into all the normal fights I would get into with a normal hearing brother, and I think I grew up the same way as if he were hearing. When I started hanging around with friends in the neighborhood, they would start asking "What is wrong with him?" And I'd say, "He's deaf and he can't hear," and they would say, "Oh." When we would play baseball and things, they could see that there was nothing wrong with him, so they just accepted him. I think the biggest thing was that he didn't go to school around here. And so my friends across town didn't know him and I think he began to feel left out. He had no friends here and it was mainly the social thing that made us drift apart. He'd come home from school and I would go off with my friends and he would stay home alone. Because there was no one else around.

D.L.: Were you embarrassed by him?

Michael: No. Because he was accepted and I never really had to defend him, because nobody ever made fun of him around me that I know of. The only real difference was when we were playing outside, Mom would yell, "Sara, Lynda, Michael, get Robert."

I remember one thing that was different. When you were watching TV or on holidays, when you were talking with the whole family. That's a big thing with him. When you were watching a program he would say "What did he say? What did he say?" Twenty times during a half-hour program. I'd just make something up or tell him to shut up.

Jean: Now it's okay because we have captions, but I always thought the kids were mean to him. They told him to shut up because "we can't hear it."

D.L.: So who would interpret for him?

Jean: The mother. I did a lot of interpretation for him. I did an A number-one job interpreting for everything. The TV, everything in life. And even on the holidays, I do the best I can.

Paul: Robert has said he feels left out on holidays. Everyone is around talking and he is left out.

Jean: I really feel it for him, and he's told me that he hates holidays because we have lots of company on holidays and he can't follow all the conversation.

Paul: I found out what that was like. I went down to visit him at Gallaudet. Everybody was going around signing and I couldn't sign. I was the one who was left out.

Jean: We haven't learned sign language. We went for a couple of years. We were very unsuccessful at it because we just didn't work at it long enough. And so we don't know sign language and Robert doesn't use sign language around us at all because none of us know it. This weekend he had a couple of friends over from Gallaudet and one was very oral. The other couldn't lipread or speak, and I felt really bad that I didn't take it. I guess that's another thing I wish I had done. And I don't know if I'll do it, yet.

Paul: But at the time when we were going through, everything was oral. We didn't learn to sign.

Michael: That's the first thing everybody asks me in school. Whenever I mention I have a deaf brother, they always ask do I know sign language. I say "No." And then they say "How do you talk to him?" I just tell them he reads lips.

Jean: He is a good lipreader and I think it's been good because at least he has to be oral around us. But I just feel badly about some of his friends who come over. He has to translate me to them. We have the TTY for him and the captioner. It's hard for him on holidays because he feels really left out of it. The talking and laughing. That's the only time I ever really feel sorry for him because he once sat down with me one day and told me how much he hates the holidays. And so that's in my head now, and every holiday that comes I feel really badly for him. I always try to tell him what's going on.

D.L.: All through his growing up, did you have that role?

Jean: Yeah, I think I had the most patience. A lot of that was from the early training of how to work with a deaf child, too. It just grew with me. And I knew I had to explain all these things to him so he would learn about them all. Television was good for him to learn but I had to sit down and tell him and explain. It was all my early training. I knew it was important for him. I think I did all that for him so that his understanding of life would be broader and he would be better for it when he grew up. And he would be able to take care of himself. Even now, even though he hasn't decided what he wants to do, I don't feel that I'll have to take care of him. I picture him, no matter what, he'll manage. That's the kind of kid he is. But I just want him to have what I want him to have in life, what I think is great. Maybe my goals are set too high; maybe that's wrong. You do that for all your kids, don't you? It's not just him.

Michael: I get frustrated now because I don't think he can lipread as good now as he could before, with all the signing. I get frustrated trying to tell him things.

Jean: You never made any concessions because he was deaf. *Michael*: No. I would yell at him. I don't know why. It was just the frustration.

D.L.: How do you think the deafness changed the family?

Jean: Well, at different stages. I guess the biggest change was when he was little and he took up so much time and energy. We didn't have a normal existence. Having to go into Boston, having to get babysitters. We were so involved in it. I was so tired. It took a lot of wear and tear and it continued until he got out of high school. I had to take him to sports and other things and it tied me up. Stress and worry, all the different turmoil in all the different school programs, always wondering if we made the right decisions. I spent a lot of nights awake trying to figure this out, because I'm one of those people who worries about everything. When he went away to college, it was like they say, "Out of sight, out of mind." He'd call me up and I'd start worrying again. But that was the most relaxing time, when he was at Gallaudet. And even now, it's relaxing until he comes home on the weekends. He keeps emotions high.

Paul: I don't think his deafness changed our life that much. Everything in the family went on just the same. We wouldn't do anything else that we didn't do. We always went on vacation. We didn't change our lifestyle.

Jean: As I think back on it, he wasn't anymore of a problem than any of the other kids. He was a pain in the neck and a hard kid to bring up. But they were kid problems, it wasn't really because he was deaf. I don't think any of us in the family ever was ashamed of him. Because no matter where you went, he always stood out in a crowd and made everyone laugh. He had a very popular personality, so we never had any problems in that way. He could do everything well and he could play all the games very well. And he was a good athlete.

Paul: His deafness probably helped him with that because he could concentrate on the games and he didn't get distracted. He did all the normal things—got his driver's license.

D.L.: So your fathering would have been the same whether he was deaf or not?

Paul: I think so. Don't you?

Jean: Yes. I think its the same with Nicole. We just treat her the same. We take her everywhere. People are more embarrassed by a retarded child than by a deaf child, but it doesn't make any difference to us. She goes to restaurants with us. We've had many occasions where people are very ignorant about things. At times, it's pretty blatant, but that is their loss, not ours.

Paul: With Robert, it's an unseen handicap. Nothing shows. With Nicole, it's something that shows.

D.L.: Were you embarrassed by Nicole?

Paul: No.

Jean: With Nicole we have had real problems in the neighborhood with very ignorant parents who won't let their children play with her for fear that she would hurt them. Robert was always accepted in the neighborhood. And even if he didn't have the kids outside, he had the members of the family. Nicole has no one. Our problems are bigger with the outside world but she is much easier to get along with.

D.L.: What was the source of your support?

Jean: Well, I don't think there was anything. Just bringing him to these programs and talking to people, and reading books. The best suport we got was in the Emerson program. It was the parent group. It was a real supportive thing. I wish we had it for Nicole. The other parents were always our biggest support. These people are stil our friends. Most of our friends have handicapped children.

Paul: With anything, it's knowing you are not alone. That's the whole thing. Being able to share your experiences.

D.L.: How about the grandparents?

Jean: Paul's parents died when Robert was very young. They just felt sorry for him. My parents are the same way. It used to be "It's poor Robert." Yet now they have seen him grow and they have seen him do things and they feel very proud of him. In the beginning years, it was all sympathy, and my mother worries too much. I never liked burdening my mother or dad with more worries. I could never go to her.

D.L.: So you supported her.

Jean: Yeah, and that has been difficult through the years. I have one sister and we weren't close when Robert was young, so I had no family for support.

D.L.: So it was just the two of you.

Paul: More or less we were against the world. You just go on. You have to. There is nothing else to do. Jeanie had more of the burden than I did. She was here and had to be here. I could escape to my work every day.

Jean: Tell him how you felt about when I was all burdened and I got frustrated and angry and sick and tired of it all, and maybe let it out on you. How did you feel about that?

Paul: Well, I think I understood. Did I fail you?

Jean: I can remember only good. I can remember when Nicole was born, I really felt awful. Yet, I think it was because of Robert. He was 12 at the time and still involved in lots of problems. It was like having to start out again, and I didn't think I could do it. I think for the first four months, Paul just kept me alive. Because I just didn't want to face it. Everybody wanted me to meet people, like other parents of Down's syndrome children, and I didn't want to see anyone. It was only Paul saying we could do it. I knew a lot of it was I just broke down from Robert, and here we go again. That was one of the effects of the deafness.

D.L.: You just fell apart.

Jean: Yeah. I just went through everything in those four months that I had gone through in the 12 years of Robert. It was going to be worse, because I didn't know what Down's syndrome was, and from what I was reading, it was very derogatory, all very down. I was just thinking the worst: I had only remembered seeing institutionalized children with Down's Syndrome. It was very tough.

Paul: It was the second time. It was starting over again.

D.L.: It looks like Paul was your sole support.

Jean: Very definitely. He was my complete strength. I just fell apart.

D.L.: Did you have that role with Robert?

Paul: I don't think so. Not at that time. I don't think we thought deafness was so bad. We just didn't think about it. We were so busy.

Jean: They were two different things. With Nicole, we knew at birth. It was like a death. The death of a dream in a way. With Robert, we didn't have to go through any of that, because we had a little time to adjust. We were really thankful when they told us he was deaf because now we could get to work at it. We knew something was wrong. Nicole was much harder to take.

D.L.: You guys have been twice bitten.

Jean: It was more than that. Lynda was born with a form of spinal bifida and when she was in the fifth grade, she had to have her spine fused. Fortunately, everything worked well, but she was traumatized by the hospital and she had a lot of trouble in school. She was the one who was most affected by Robert's deafness. She used to cry everytime we left her. We were just not affected by the deafness because we didn't have any time to dwell on it. Now I look back on it, I don't know how I could have done it.

D.L.: Do you see any good come out of this?

Jean: We met a lot of nice people.

Paul: Yeah, we sure did.

Jean: It's been interesting, really. There have been a lot of good things.

Paul: Yeah, a lot of awareness of things around a lot of different kinds of people.

Jean: I think my kids were really good because of it, too. They were much more sensitive to other people's feelings. They spoke out about things, and I think that was a good thing, too.

Michael: I think I would have been more critical of other people, especially in a town like this. For example, a black family moved down the street, and they ran them out of town. This town is sort of prejudiced.

Jean: Yeah. None of us is prejudiced. We have seen so many different kinds of people.

Michael: It educated us as far as retarded people and deaf people.

D.L.: How did it affect your marriage?

Paul: I think it brought us closer together, because we did things together. We probably wouldn't have otherwise.

Jean: I think the same thing. Paul, to me, has never been somebody who, if something is bothering him—who needs somebody to talk to about it. He just keeps everything in. But I am a very talkative person and I need someone to talk to, and it's nice to have someone to listen.

We have lots of friends who have problems in their marriage because one person wouldn't accept it. Paul never had a macho thing even though I had German measles and my age when I had Nicole. Neither one of us ever laid a guilt trip on the other. We each felt we had to take the ball and run with it because this is what you got.

Paul: I was amazed to find among the parents of the school for the deaf how many broken families there were. I didn't know if it was because of the deafness, but I was amazed.

D.L.: If you had it to do over again, what would you do differently?

Paul: Well, first, I think Jean and I both agree on this. We pushed him to go to Gallaudet. I wished he went to a technical school. And I think we would have kept him back one year. We pushed him but he wasn't very mature. He graduated high school when he was 18.

Jean: That's true. It wasn't so much pushing. We gave him a lot of therapy and he did very well. But maybe we should have said, "I think he is immature." Academically, he was ahead of everyone. I think that's the mistake we made, because maturity is just as important as academics, and we weren't thinking that way at all.

There was also all of that turmoil at the high school. They were having meetings to get rid of people, and Robert needed something normal going on. That was a mess. We made so many changes; maybe that wasn't good either. Although I don't know what we could have done because the day class programs were not very good, and there had to be a change.

D.L.: It sounds like when he's here, there's a lot more tension and stress in the family?

Jean: There's just something about Robert! It's just something about him. When we see his car drive up we say, "Here he comes!" The tension just goes up. I don't feel sorry for Robert. I feel sorry for us. The minute he comes in he has to tease Nicole. He's the biggest tease—I can't believe it—and he's also a lot of fun, and has given us some very proud days too.

D.L.: Do you feel good about your family?

Jean: I do. I think when they were growing up I thought of all the things I figured I was doing wrong, but now that I see the outcome of it all, I really do feel that everything turned out pretty well. They are all very nice kids. And I think I was a good wife and a good mother. There was a lot of success there. I didn't always think so but I have matured through the years, too.

D.L.: Do you feel good about them too, Paul?

Paul: Yeah. As Jean says, the same thing. They are good happy people and really making their way in the world.

At my request Sara and Lynda Murphy wrote of their recollections of the family.

Dear Dr. Luterman:
I have been very busy this spring with work, my two special education classes that I am taking at the University of Hawaii, and the new group that I joined called *Sign Express*. It is a group of about 15 people that sign songs and put on performances to help educate others about sign language.
I am real excited, about the book you are writing and I wish that I could have been there to talk with you when you went over to my family's house. I have a lot of feelings about Robert's deafness and how it has affected me. I have only told my mother some of my feelings because she gets upset or angry when I say how I felt when I was little. I don't know if it is because she thinks that I am saying that she was not a good mother to me, or why she gets upset.
I think when I was little, I had very mixed feelings. I felt very jealous of Robert but I also felt very proud of him. I can remember feeling very neglected, because I always thought that he got all of the attention from everybody. Of course, now I realize that my mother had to work with him more and it was all necessary, but I didn't understand that when I was little. I remember wishing that I was deaf for a while thinking that then I would get more attention. I remember wishing that I would get sick and have to go into the hospital so that everyone would bring me presents and give me more attention. I even remember trying to break my arm by jumping out of my treehouse (which never happened). I have never told my mother any of this. But I never hated Robert. I guess the way I dealt with my jealousy was by deciding to work with deaf children when I grew up. I decided this ever since I used to go watch Robert at Emerson College through the one-way mirror with my mother. And here I am, a speech pathologist working at a school where the deaf total communication class is housed, and I love working with the deaf kids (ages 5–12).
I also remember being very proud of Robert. I can remember going to his school plays at the school for the deaf and having tears come to my eyes when I watched him on stage. I remember wanting to be friends with his friends there. I also remember people saying mean things about deaf people in general, like they can't talk and they are all "deaf and dumb," and feeling so hurt and intimidated that I couldn't even stand up for deaf people. I usually just said nothing.
I guess Robert's deafness probably created a lot of extra tension in

my parents' marriage. I remember my mother getting really upset about the taxis taking him to school, some school problem, and other things. I remember my father not wanting or just not getting involved and my mother getting upset at him. I really never understood just how it affected my father but I know it was real hard on my mother. I never really noticed what affect Robert's deafness had on Lynda, Michael, or Nicole. I didn't get along with Lynda, Michael, or Robert that much when I was little.

Now I am much closer to everyone in my family. Maybe it's because I live so far away. I am trying to learn to sign fluently. Robert prefers to sign now and doesn't associate with hearing people if he can help it. Last summer, when I went home for a visit, I played the card game Uno with Robert and his friends. At first I felt uncomfortable, but it was a lot of fun and I think that was the first time anyone in our family associated with him when he had his friends over. I wish I could spend more time with him and really get to know him. I have been able to get a hold of a TTY a few times and I love being able to talk to him over the phone. I always felt bad when I called home on holidays and could talk to everyone and then just be able to tell someone to say hi to Robert. I remember a couple of times he would get on the phone to say hi to me and then my mother would get on the phone and say "that was Robert," like I couldn't tell. I remember when we used to watch TV when we were little and Robert would always ask us what was going on in the show and we would get so irritated at him and tell him to wait for the commercials. I wish we knew how to sign then and be able to interpret for him so he could understand while the show was on. I have very strong feelings about total communication. Robert has told me a lot about how he always felt left out and that makes me feel so sad for him because if we only used sign language he would have been more involved and would have known what was going on. But I realize that is a big issue that probably never will be solved.

Well I guess I rambled on quite a bit. I hope that this information will be helpful to you. If you have any more questions, please feel free to write to me. I'll be glad to help in any way possible. I would love to visit you the next time I get back to Boston and also visit the clinic at Emerson College. Thank you for asking my feelings.

Sincerely,
Sara Murphy

Dear Dr. Luterman:
As far as Robert's deafness having an effect on me, I see mostly positive things. He has a very strong character as well as personality, so I've never felt sorry for him. Of course, I wish he wasn't deaf, but that's beside the point. There is one incident that does stand out in my memory. I'll never forget it. My whole family was vacationing in Washington, D.C. I was 13 so Robert would have been 11. We were waiting

for a tour to start and I was sitting next to Robert talking with him. There was a woman next to him and she asked me what was wrong with him, I told her that he was deaf. I never saw him so upset. He was absolutely infuriated with me. He ran off and when I caught up told me. He said he was mad that I told that lady he was deaf (he didn't see her ask me what was wrong with him) because he said he didn't like people to know because they would look at him funny. When I told him that she had asked me because of his speech, he was shocked. He really had no idea that his voice or speech was any different than mine or yours. When I thought about it later, as I did many times, I was ashamed to have embarrassed him over something that we just assumed he realized.

I remember having to stamp on the floor to get his attention if he was across the room and how mad I used to get at him for closing his eyes when I was arguing with him. I think that our family should be proud of how well adjusted he is and really always has been. He was always comfortable around my friends, although he would get frustrated when they would have to look at me for translation more often than not. What I think is important is that he was frustrated and not embarrassed. As he got into junior high and high school, it seemed to be a whole new lifestyle for him. He was using sign language almost exclusively, except with us at home, since none of us knew it. He had joined a deaf club and got his drivers license, got a speeding ticket, got drunk for the first time (don't tell my Mom), and was just a normal teenager. It had finally come full circle when he had some friends over and he introduced me to them and they proceeded to sign to each other and looked at me and laughed. I thought "Now I know what it feels like to be in a room where people are talking and I don't know what they're saying." It was a very strange feeling. I plan to enroll in a sign language class this fall so that I can be involved with his friends just as he always tried to be and was with mine. I love Robert very much and have always been proud of him, never embarrassed by him. I hope I've helped you and I anxiously await the book!

Sincerely,
Lynda Murphy

This family's coping strategy was to leave it all to the mother/wife. She was clearly given a great deal of emotional support by her husband and a great deal of positive reinforcement for her mothering. This apparently enabled her to be a positive parent. It served also to strengthen greatly the mother-child bond, so that Jean became Robert's interpreter and his primary teacher. This is a frequent outcome of a parent education program that evolves into a mother-education program. She was greatly burdened by the task; although it was one that she willingly undertook, seeing it as her responsibility to raise her children. Paul's responsibility was to be the breadwinner and supporter of Jean. At times, Jean wanted more, but the roles were pretty rigidly prescribed in this family, and there did not appear to be much room for change. Jean has done a remarkable job, at one point having had four children under the age of 5, with a very difficult deaf child to raise. That she did this, and remained sane in the process, is a testimony to her strength. The incredible feat she pulled off was not always appreciated by professionals and is only beginning to be appreciated by the rest of the family. On top of coping with Robert's many problems, she also had to deal with Lynda's medical and school difficulties. All of this with a minimum of physical support. Her one "breakdown" within the family was shortly after Nicole's birth, and that altered Paul's role markedly. In order to restore family homeostasis at that time, he had to provide much more support than he had on previous occasions, and the rigid role boundaries were breached somewhat, although now that Jean has recovered, the family paradigm of leaving the child-rearing and educational decisions to Jean has reemerged. While perhaps not an optimal situation, the family is certainly quite adequate and well on its way to fulfilling its primary mission, to produce independent adults.

Both parents are dealing with guilt. Neither is very happy with Robert's present status and they both feel that they are somehow responsible for it. I think assuming the awesome responsibility of parenthood leaves all parents vulnerable to guilt. Having a child with special needs, which means having to be a "special parent," increases enormously the opportunities for feeling guilty. It is not at all clear that the Murphys could have done anything differently. All parents want to do the right things for their children and are constrained by the limitations, of programmatic options and their own values and expectations, which very often serve as blinders.

Right now, the Murphy's are dealing with two issues concerning Robert. They are confronted with the very pressing affiliation issue, Robert's preference for the "deaf world" and the family exclusion from that world, as well as Robert's exclusion from much of the family's life. The family has not evolved any good solution for this problem; no one still living at home has learned sign language—they haven't felt the need to because of his good oral skills—and Robert is unwilling to stay within a hearing framework, where he is clearly uncomfortable. I think this can only lead to further estrangement.

It is tempting to see this problem as solely one of disrupted communication due to the deafness, that if the family would learn sign language many of their communicaton problems would disappear. I don't think this is true at all. Communication with a teenager is tenuous at best, whether or not he or she can hear. In my experience, families who use total communication are not any better off than families of children who are oral. Most hearing parents do not develop sufficient manual communication skills to communicate fully with their child in the complexity needed to negotiate with a teenager. Swisher and Thompson (1985) found that hearing mothers of children of approximately 5 years of age who had three years of training in sign language signed only 40 percent of the spoken utterance to their children. My clinical experience is that, as the child gets older, parents fall further behind in their manual communication skills and are far outstripped by their child who uses it intensively every day and acquires new vocabulary in school. The parents, meanwhile, usually have stopped going to sign classes, and the only practice they get is with their child. Their skills generally atrophy and stagnate, since they get such limited use. I doubt that, if Jean and Paul were to learn sign language, any of their current problems with Robert would disappear. Almost all the families I know with a deaf child must continually strive to overcome a communication gap in addition to the generation gap. This communication gap is present whether or not they use manual communication.

The second issue that the family is currently concerned with is Robert's leaving home. To the parents the present situation is unsatisfactory; it seems a partial solution at best to the final break that all children must make. The family's homeostasis is clearly disrupted every weekend when he returns from his job. I think it very likely that tensions are building in this family to such a degree that a major change is bound to take place soon.

Robert Murphy's view:

I don't know what to say first, but I remember I had a very happy childhood and growing up years. I felt my family was very good to me. They cared about me very much and gave me a lot of love. That's very important. We communicated in oralism. We didn't have much trouble. If they didn't understand me or I didn't understand they would finger spell or have the patience to repeat. It was not a problem that they knew no sign language.

My neighborhood was very good to me. They treated me very nice. I was close to my mother and my brother. I remember my mother told me about being deaf but that I was very special and that made me feel very good. I remember, when I came home from school, my Mom always asked me what I did in school. She always like [sic] to help and encourage me with my schoolwork. I felt that I learned a lot from her and she has a gift to raise me very well and I felt that, no wonder God gave us another handicapped child [Nicole].

My brother was great to me, also. I was very happy to have a brother like him. I always played with him and always have [sic] fun but, of course, sometime [sic] fight, too.

If I didn't have Michael I wouldn't have had many friends around the neighborhood and also being a good athlete [sic].

My dad and I didn't have too much of a relationship. My dad was always very busy, but I remember my dad helped me in sports. He always attend [sic] all baseball and hockey and swim events. He also was a coach for me on baseball and assistant coach later on. I remember I was in a slump in baseball and my dad was angry at me so he took me to a field and worked hard to help me out of my slump. It worked! I wish we had more time together.

My oldest sister Sara liked to play with me and I also remember I didn't like to be near her because she was so mushy to me!! She now knows sign language and works with deaf people [children].

Lynda was the most patient person. She was always willing to take time to focus on me and help explain. She always makes me laugh.

Nicole is a great, lovable sister to me. I felt it is great to have a younger sister. I learned how to take care of children with her. I remembered the day she was born, my dad told me it was a girl and I was disappointed because I wanted a brother, but when I saw her in the hospital I was very thrilled! I remember my dad an [sic] Susan tryed [sic] to explain to me what Down's syndrome is. I read books. It was a little scary but when my mom brought Nicole home it wasn't scary anymore and now she is very smart and sweet and I love to be with her.

I remember going to nursery school at Emerson College. I loved playing and seeing Santa Claus.

I went to seven different schools, all around and all different. It wasn't so bad except for taxi's [sic] because my Mom always cheered me up. After mainstreaming in the beginning, I was happy to go to a school for the deaf. I saw so many kids with hearing aids and had so many peers, then to mainstream high school. I was involved in swimming and had many friends, hearing and deaf. I went to Gallaudet for two years but it didn't work out for me. I really still don't know about my future. I'm working now to find out.

My social life now is very good. I'm very involved with the Deaf Community. I prefer to be social with the Deaf because it is easier to communicate, but I have many hearing friends, too.

In the future, I know I will always be close to my family. I look at my past and it was wonderful but right now I have a lot of big decisions to make and it is tough. My parents want me to get a degree but I still have to decide what to major in. I'm looking forward to making all my family proud of me even prouder than they are already.

REFERENCE

Swisher, M. V., & Thompson, M. (1985). Mothers learning simultaneous communication: The dimensions of the task. *American Annals of the Deaf, 130,* 212–216.

CHAPTER 5

Siblings

Siblings form the first social laboratory for the individual's experiments with peer relationships. Within the sibling system, children can learn how to resolve conflicts and support one another. They learn how to negotiate among equals or near equals. (They learn how to deal with authority in their relationships with their parents.) The sibling system teaches them how to make friends and allies, how to save face while losing, and how to achieve recognition for their skills. In the sibling world, children learn how to negotiate, cooperate, and compete. The jockeying for position within the family system shapes and molds children into their adult roles. When children come into contact with the world outside the family, they take with them the knowledge they learned from their siblings to form their peer relationships. "Children who have no siblings tend to develop an early pattern of accommodation to the adult world which is seen at first as precocious social development. These children, however, have difficulty in the development of autonomy and in the ability to share, cooperate, and compete with others" (Minuchin, 1974).

It is not clear from an examination of the rather sparse literature as to what happens to the sibling subsystem when a handicapped child is introduced into the family. In the Wagner family, both Conrad and Kate felt that Laura was "different" and "special" and neither would fight as long or as hard with her as they would with each other. This might be a function of the message sent by their parents that Laura was somehow more delicate than anyone else; or it might be, as Kate said, that it was just too hard to explain to her what was going on, so you did not play the practical joke or prolong the argument any longer than necessary. One wonders not only how this affected Kate and Conrad, but also Laura, who was not given a good opportunity to learn conflict resolution skills.

The Murphy family, on the other hand, seemed to make no concessions to Robert's deafness. He and Michael had many fights and Michael feels that the deafness made no difference in their conflicts and in the family's treatment of Robert. There appears to be a very close sibling subsystem in the Murphy family, with only a five year spread among the four older children. This sibling subsystem pretty much had to function on its own and was the primary socialization vehicle for the children.

Probably the most definitive study of siblings in the literature of the handicapped was conducted by Grossman (1972). She tested and interviewed in depth 83 college students who had retarded siblings. Some subjects were selected from a prestigious private university and the others from a community college. She found that 45 percent of the subjects benefited from the retarded sibling, 45 percent were harmed, and 10 percent were not affected. Those not affected by the presence of the retarded sibling in the family tended to be older brothers, who were often exempt from any physical care responsibilities. Those most affected were the oldest sisters, who were expected to participate in child-rearing activities and to assume many parental functions. There were very different role expectations for oldest sons than for oldest daughters. All younger silbings were affected one way or the other by the retarded child.

The negative consequences noted by Grossman were
1. Shame about the retarded child, then guilt about the shame.
2. Guilt about being in good health.
3. A sense of being tainted or defective; concern about whether they themselves might be retarded or might bear retarded children.
4. Guilt about having negative feelings towards the retarded sibling.
5. A feeling of having been neglected by their parents.
6. A feeling of having lost their own childhood because of the early assumption of responsibilities.
7. A belief that the retarded child had put a stress on the parental relationship, which negatively affected the rest of the family.

The positives in the situation were seen as
1. Greater understanding of people in general and handicapped people in particular.

2. More compassion.
3. More appreciation of their own good health and intelligence.
4. More sensitivity to prejudice.
5. A sense that the experience had drawn the family together.
6. A sense of vocational purpose and direction.

As one might fully expect, Grossman found the the more open and comfortable the parents seemed to have been in talking about the retarded child's handicap, the better able the normal sibling was to deal with it. When the parents accepted the handicapped child, they tended to help the normal child come to a healthy acceptance of the retarded child. This finding has strong clinical implications for professionals working with handicapped children; by working with the parents, as systems theory would predict, they also are working with the sibling system. The other finding that needs to be emphasized is that, as tragic as having a handicapped child may be, it can and does have a very positive effect on some families.

Several further studies of siblings of handicapped children reported in the literature support Grossman's findings of both positive and negative effects. For example, Gath (1973) found that more antisocial behavior was reported in sisters of children with Down's syndrome than in a matched control group. Trevino (1979), reviewing literature on siblings of handicapped children, concluded that the siblings are potentially at risk and early identification is essential to aid in the alleviation of the adverse effects.

On the other hand, Cleveland and Miller (1977) obtained responses to a questionnaire by 90 siblings of institutionalized retarded adults. They found that the majority of the normal siblings felt that they had a positive adaptation to the retarded child. Sisters tended to choose helping careers more often than brothers, the sisters who seemed to suffer some adverse effects were the only or oldest girl in the family.

Breslau, Weitzman, and Messenger (1981) compared 239 normal siblings (ages 6–18) of children with cystic fibrosis, cerebral palsy, myelodysplasia, and multiple handicapping conditions with a control group of siblings of nonhandicapped children. Results of the study indicated that, as a group, siblings of handicapped children did not differ from the control siblings in overall psychological functioning. Seligman (1983), after an extensive review of the literature, concluded that there is a differential effect, noting that the preponderance of studies present a pessimistic view of the effect on siblings. Vadasy, Fewell, Meyer, and Schell (1984) and Lobato (1983) call for longitudinal and better controlled observational studies of families, so as to increase the understanding of how children adapt to a sibling's handicaps. I fully concur with this need.

There are only two studies on the siblings of deaf children, both of which can be considered as preliminary attempts in an area that needs considerable exploration. Schwirian (1976) interviewed 29 mothers of families in which there was a preschool hearing-impaired child with older siblings. She devised a structured interview schedule that measured a Child Care Index (the extent to which the sibling was responsible for the hearing-impaired child), a Responsibility Index (responsibility for general household duties), an Independence Index (how much freedom was granted the sibling), and a Social Activity Index (the number of close friends the child had). She had a control group of 28 families with only normal-hearing children. Schwirian found that the older hearing siblings of hearing-handicapped preschool children had greater child care responsibilities and less social activities (fewer friends) than the control group who had normally hearing siblings. Sisters had significantly higher child care and overall responsibility scores than brothers, again indicating the different role expectation that parents have for sons and daughters. She found, however, that the four areas of behavior were influenced more by the age and sex of the subject than by any of the other independent variables, regardless of the presence of the hearing-impaired child. In short, she was unable to tease from her data any statistically significant effect that could be attributed directly to the presence of a hearing-impaired child in the family. It must be noted that, in this study, there was no direct observation or testing of the subjects. All of the data were obtained through interviews with the mothers. The mothers, however, may not have a very clear idea of what the siblings are experiencing; witness, for example, Sara Murphy's inability to talk about her feelings with her mother.

Israelite (1986), on the other hand, tested 14 hearing female adolescents (mean age, 16 years 3 months), who were the older sisters of hearing-impaired children, and a matched control group of 14 adolescents who had hearing siblings, on four test measures: the Family Responsibility Index (adapted from the Schwirian study), Beck Depression Inventory, Speilberger State-Trait Anxiety Inventory, and the Tennessee Self-Concept Scale. All these tests are self-report questionnaires. She found that the sisters of hearing-impaired children differed significantly on only two traits, self-concept–identity and social self. The results suggested that the hearing siblings defined themselves not only as individuals in their own right, but as sisters of hearing-impaired children. It is problemmatic as to how much this affected their social life. There were no significant differences between the groups on the measures of family responsibility, depression, anxiety, and self-esteem.

I think that the effects of the hearing-impaired child on the hearing sibling are both subtle and variable, in large part, depending on the parents' ability to cope with the problem and the speed and sensitivity with which professional help is available to the family. What is needed badly at this point is a large scale, Grossman-type study, in which the siblings are both tested and interviewed in depth, in order to tease out the effects of the deaf siblings on the hearing children. The measures used by both Schwirian and Israelite were crude and their samples of subjects were very limited. Both investigators also assumed that the effects of the deaf child in the family would be negative. This is not born out by the Grossman study data nor by my own observations of families. I think there can be a very positive effect on the siblings as well as increased stress. Conrad and Kate Wagner, for example, felt that Laura made them more aware and sensitive to other people and to the handicapped in particular. They both felt that their priorities were shaped very positively by Laura's deafness. Michael Murphy felt he was much less prejudiced and was broadened by his early exposure to deafness and retardation; both he and his oldest sister, Sara, are involved in special education, which is a direct reflection of their family life, I think.

Systems theory would predict that normal siblings would also have an effect on the impaired child; that there would be a bidirectional flow of effect. I have been unable to find any studies to document how the presence of hearing siblings affects the hearing-impaired child. One could predict that deaf children from families with hearing siblings would have greater socialization skills and better speech and language skills than deaf children with no hearing siblings. It is not uncommon, for example, for parents to use an older, hearing sibling as a surrogate therapist, and he or she always provides a role model of speech and language use and a peer with which the deaf child can practice communication. For example, Kate and Conrad had some responsibility for teaching Laura words. I think the hearing sibling, if his or her needs are well met and if used well by parents and professionals, can be a potent help in the habilitation of the hearing-impaired child. Clearly, this is a rich, untapped area for research.

I think the feelings of the siblings are very similar to the parental feelings. In fact, the siblings take their cues from the parents. They have many fears related to their own hearing and to their own vulnerability. Having a deaf sibling increases their social isolation and loneliness. They now somehow are different from their peers. Conrad and Kate, for example, were reluctant to bring friends home because of the awkwardness of the friends first encounters with Laura. They also had an identity that was different from anyone else's.

Anger is often present, stemming from many different sources. Some arise from the normal sibling socialization kinds of conflict. Other angers emerge from the frustration of communication and the misunderstandings due to the deafness. Frequently, anger or resentment is born out of the increased attention that the deaf child demands and receives from the parents and other significant relatives. There is an anger about assuming caretakerlike functions sooner than they would have liked. Almost all hearing siblings have to assume some responsibility for the deficiencies of the deaf child; for example, the older sister who tutors her younger, mainstreamed brother in most of his school subjects or the younger sibling who answers the phone and makes calls for an older hearing-impaired sibling. These increased responsibilities can be seen as just something one does and is accepted with a shrug, or they can be fraught with much resentment. Again, it is a matter of the family paradigm around the deafness, and in particular, in the way in which the parents accept and deal with their own increased responsibilities.

Almost all hearing siblings feel some guilt that they can hear and their sibling cannot. This guilt very often holds them back from engaging fully in the give and take of sibling conflict. There also is increased pressure on the siblings to perform better to compensate for the parental "failure" and their sibling's inadequacies. This effect, noted by Featherstone (1980) in her family, is common in families with a deaf child.

None of these feelings need have a negative effect on the siblings, if they are dealt with well by the parents. There needs to be an openness within the families so that information is conveyed to the siblings and there are adequate outlets for the expression of feelings. Decisions that will effect everyone in the family must be discussed. The sibling needs to feel that his or her needs are being considered as well and that he or she is important within the family.

The family position of the sibling is also an important variable. I think the Grossman finding also is true for deaf families: the oldest sisters are given more caretaking responsibilities and are more affected by their sibling's deafness than older brothers or other older sisters. This is especially true in lower socioeconomic levels, where there tend to be more sex role stereotyping and less financial resources to buy caretaking services than in higher socioeconomic levels. I think it is clear in the Murphy family that Sara has been affected by Robert's deafness more so than Michael or Lynda.

Where the deaf child is the oldest child, as in the Wagner family, the hearing sibling becomes a reminder, sometimes painful, of the extent of the disability. The younger child also helps to keep the disability in perspective. One is reminded of the Wagners sitting outside Kate's door listening to her babble and thinking what a miracle that was. Parents with younger, hearing children frequently remark that they never realized how easy it is to bring up a hearing child and how easy communication is. My own impression is that in families where the deaf child is born first followed by hearing siblings who are close in age, the deaf child is allowed much more freedom and tends to be more independent. The parents simply cannot afford to be too protective of the deaf child. In families in which the deaf child is the youngest, that child tends to be more dependent and more restricted by both the parents and older siblings, who assume caretaker roles. For example, Robert's difficulty in separating and assuming responsiblity for himself may be directly, related to his position as the youngest child for a long time; while Laura Wagner, as the oldest child, is clearly better prepared to be an independent adult.

Another variable that has not been looked at extensively is family size. One could predict that in larger families there would be less of a negative effect on any one sibling, because there would be a number of siblings to share the burden. Grossman (1972) found this to be so with the oldest sisters of retarded children; oldest siblings from larger families coped better with their sibling's retardation than siblings from smaller families. There is no information about the impact of family size on a deaf child.

Obviously, a multitude of variables affect the siblings in the family, and it is very hard to pinpoint any one variable. Family size, sex of siblings, age differences among siblings, and socioeconomic status of the family all seem to play roles. Of enormous significance is how well the parents manage their own feelings and their child management skills determining whether the siblings benefit or are harmed by the deaf sibling. There seems to be a complex interplay among all of the variables and few persons emerge from the family unscathed.

As a profession, I think we have begun to respond to the feelings of the deaf individuals and their parents. However, we have not listened to the feelings of the hearing siblings. Sara Murphy poignantly thanks me for asking about her feelings. I think the hearing siblings have been neglected far too long.

REFERENCES

Breslau, N., Weitzman, M., & Messenger, K. (1981). Psychologic functioning of siblings of disabled children. *Pediatrics, 67,* 344–353.

Cleveland, D. W., & Miller, N. (1977). Attitudes and life commitments of older siblings of mentally retarded adults. *Mental Retardation, 15,* 38–41.

Featherstone, H. (1980). *A Difference in the family: Living with a disabled child.* New York: Basic Books.

Gath, A. (1973). The school age siblings of mongol children. *Social Casework: The Journal of Contemporary Social Work, 60,* 488–493.

Grossman, F. K. (1972). *Brothers and sisters of retarded children.* Syracuse, NY: Syracuse University Press.

Israelite, N. K. (1986). Hearing-impaired children and the psychological functioning of their normal hearing siblings. *Volta Review, 88,* 47–54.

Lobato, D., (1983). Siblings of handicapped children: A review. *Journal of Autism and Developmental Disorders, 13,* 347–364.

Minuchin, S. (1974). *Families and family therapy.* Cambridge, MA: Harvard University Press.

Schwirian, P. (1976). Effects of the presence of a hearing-impaired preschool child in the family on behavior patterns of older "normal" siblings. *American Annals of the Deaf, 121,* 373–380.

Seligman, M. (1983). Siblings of handicapped persons. In M. Seligman (Ed.), *The family with a handicapped child: Understanding and treatment.* New York: Grune and Stratton.

Trevino, F. (1979). Siblings of handicapped children: Identifying those at risk. *Social Casework: The Journal of Contemporary Social Work, 60,* 488–493.

Vadasy, P., Fewell, R., Meyer, D., & Schell, G. (1984). Siblings of handicapped children: A developmental perspective on family interactions. *Family Relations, 33,* 155–167.

CHAPTER 6

Family in Practice:
The Marshalls

Bob Marshall, a computer programmer age 45, is currently planning to start his own company. His wife Susan, a trained nurse age 42, recently obtained a degree in psychology. Susan has worked periodically on a parttime basis in addition to going to school. The Marshalls have three children. The oldest, Nancy, 19, is deaf; she is attending a small liberal arts college in New England. Andrew, a normally hearing child age 18, is a senior in their local high school. Eighteen months ago he was involved in a serious car accident in which he sustained leg and head injuries from which he is still recovering. His parents discovered that he had been having problems with alcohol and drugs; and he is currently attending a rehabilitation program. The youngest child, Timothy, 16, also is deaf and is mainstreamed in the local high school.

D.L.: Can you tell me about your family history?

Susan: When Nancy was 12 months old, Andrew was born. I was taking Nancy to the pediatrician for a physical. Bob's mother called the pediatrician and said, "I'm not sure but I don't think Nancy is hearing well." She would say to me, "Gee, Nancy doesn't seem to know her name," but because this was my first child and I thought that Nancy heard, I really didn't know what my mother-in-law meant. So, when we went to the pediatrician, he clapped his hands several times and she turned around. He told us to watch her during the next week, so we began testing her but she didn't respond, so the pediatrician sent us to Children's Hospital. I remember sitting in the waiting room listening to the audiologist explain to another family that their child had a nerve deafness. That was the first time it occurred to me that Nancy could be deaf. After they tested her in that little room, he came out and said, "Well, your daughter is probably deaf and she will never talk right and never hear." That was devastating. I remember we got hearing aids and then we went to Emerson. I was in a fog. We were looking at Andrew and he seemed fine. Then Timothy came along two years later and he definitely did hear, but for two years his hearing fluctuated. He'd hear for one week and then he wouldn't hear for a few weeks. So I was bringing him around to all these doctors and he had fluid in his ears. Finally, I got a doctor to put tubes in his ears and they were finally clear, but he still couldn't hear well. One Memorial Day weekend, when he was 2 years old, he "turned off" and it never came back. He started wearing two hearing aids, and a few years later complained that one aid was not working. It was found that he has no usable hearing in that ear. He has a 75–85 dB loss in the other ear. And Nancy has a 95 dB loss in both ears.

After Emerson, Nancy went to a local nursery school and, at the same time, to a day class program within our school system. She started kindergarten here and has gone through the system. Timothy has done the same thing. Nancy repeated the third grade and I'm not sure she needed to. In grammar school, she would go one period a day to see the teacher of the deaf. Once she got to high school, she had an aide in a few of her classes who would help her. Timothy spent two years in the first grade and he's a sophomore now with an aide. He's having more trouble than Nancy. He was just tested and they found he has some learning disabilities. Every year, I have to fight with the school and arrange with the school for their programs, etc. They pay the aides peanuts. Now, with Andrew's problems, I'm always at the school. They sure know me there. You get tired of this fighting all the time.

Bob: You run out of gas.

D.L.: Is that where you are now? Sort of burnt out?

Nancy: Well, no. I went through a period of that for a couple of months this winter. I had a big folder on each kid with lists of things to do, people to call, etc., and it was a whole day of that, day after day of that to look forward to every day, you know, with three kids. I was at the point where all I was doing was crying. I knew I was depressed and I knew why I was depressed. So Bob and I went on vacation to Mexico. The two of us went away alone for the first time and it was very relaxing. I didn't think about the kids at all and the day we returned, Nancy arrived home from college and we had thought everything was fine. She had sounded so "up" on the TTY. She told us she is having social problems—no friends—and she doesn't think she can stay there the whole four years. I thought, "That's it!" I had it. I just had so many angry thoughts. I just had a whole mixed bag of feelings, but I feel that you have to give in to those feelings for a little while. Then, you have to get on and keep doing things. I think, well, you are only in this life for so many years and some day we are going to get out into a better world. That's what I believe.

D.L.: How do you look at it, Bob?

Bob: I had my crisis a few years ago when I was tired of work and the kids, and Susan told me to stop feeling sorry for myself. Nobody is going to do it for you. I think it was very fortunate we ran into you and your program. I hate to see the kids sad. I guess I hate to see them isolated. When they were young, they sort of blended in. As they get older, they get more separated and that really hurts. They are missing so much not talking on the phone like other teenagers. They all are great kids. They are sort of naive, like kids should be.

Susan: It's easier for Bob. He's away all day. The kids have done extremely well and I am very proud of them. Both are very resourceful and talented. Yet, they still want to be able to hear and they don't fit with deaf kids and they don't fit with hearing kids. They don't catch conversation fast enough or jokes fast enough. Just so much.

D.L.: It hurts to see them left out.

Bob: Yes. I feel sad for Nancy. I know she would have liked to have been more a part of that whole high school scene. I used to chaperone dances and it was hard to see her left out.

D.L.: Do you have regrets about going the hearing route?

Susan: No. Not for our kids. Despite the socialization problem, they have turned out well. Part of this is their deafness and part of this is their personality.

Bob: I'm like that too. I don't socialize much at work either. Now we just have the last hurdle when she graduates college and gets a job. I think we have done a good job.

D.L.: How have you made your decisions about education?

Susan: Well, Bob sort of leaves it up to me. We talk about things and Bob sort of goes along. The decisions seemed easy. After we left Emerson, there was a program for deaf kids in the town and the kids have always done pretty well. Its very difficult to send a kid away to school at age 5 or 6. And it was easier for me to treat them like normal kids and they have become like that.

Bob: That's how we made all our decisions, "Let's try this and see how it works." But once you try something, you have to have the guts to say "Okay. This isn't working," and you have to do something else. We did that several times. It's a trial and error process. Nothing is black or white.

Susan: I handled the school responsibilities but when there was a big crisis, Bob would get involved. One time with the superintendent, we had a problem and he went there.

D.L.: How has this affected your marriage?

Bob: It's kind of hard to say because it's been part of our lives so much. I admire Susan so much because she has had the brunt of things. I go off to work and it's tougher on her.

D.L.: So you really got to appreciate her.

Bob: Jokingly, I tell her there is an American Express card for her and she can leave home whenever she wants to. If she ever came down the stairs with a suitcase in her hand, I would be floored but I would understand.

Susan: This was devastating for us and it isn't anything we ever wanted. I don't think any parent would. I think we have coped with it pretty well. It's pretty much involved our whole married lives since Nancy was born. It's always there. It never leaves you.

I think marriage is a lot of luck. I think when you get married you really, really don't know. You might think you know the person you are getting married to, but you don't. It just worked out well for us. We don't have to get into deep discussions about most things. We just follow along together. Don't you think so?

Bob: I think the deafness can be a catalyst to pull a marriage together or to break it apart. I think ours was a naturally strong marriage and this kind of pulled it together. I think we are a good team. She was always out there on the front line and came back and we'd talk about it. We'd dig out the data and make decisions.

Susan: Some days you'd have a good day and I'd have a bad day and we'd sort of pull each other along.

Bob: That's the other part of it. As long as one is up. The worst part is when we're both down. Then you really have to pull your bootstraps together.

Susan: When I look back on our marriage of 21 years, I look back, we had a lot of really good times with the kids, especially when they were young. The teenagers were tough. And sometimes the kids can get between you. I think that happens to a lot of families.

D.L.: What have been some of the stresses for you?

Susan: Who knows? We've always lived with it. Our big stress has been with Andrew. You feel bad sometimes. We're so used to having the kids and they really are a joy. The part that hurts is when you see something that they want to do, when you see something that's happening with other kids that's not happening with them. That's the part that hurts. I always tell my kids, ''Nancy, it's okay to feel bad about the fact that you can't do this or that you can't do that, and I wish that you could hear, but there is nothing we can do about it. Except for you to look at the good things you have done and feel proud of yourself. You are doing things that many kids can't do.''

D.L.: Can you do that for yourself?

Susan: I do that for myself. I always think of myself as a very average person. I have no particular talent, no particular anything. I'm a very average type person. And I've been given three very special kids. Sometimes I talk to God and I say, ''Why did you give these kids to me. Why didn't you give them to someone that was different,'' and so then I think, ''All right, I was given these kids and maybe this is my thing in life. Maybe this is all I'm going to do in life is to get these kids into adulthood, and maybe that is how my salvation will be measured.''

D.L.: Is that how you look at it, Bob?

Bob: I guess I don't look at it as philosophically as Susan does. I just feel that they are here and we are doing the best we can with it. And I think we are doing okay with it. Right now, I feel I'm a much better parent now than I was five years ago. I roll with the punches, with the kids, much easier. I don't take things so seriously any more. As a result, the family is more relaxed and I feel confident that they will do fine. Nothing in life is guaranteed, although some days I feel I'm being picked on.

Susan: I think it's okay to feel that way, too, with all this stuff that has been thrown on us. When I came back from that vacation I was really angry. I was angry at God and I just said, "Look, I'm really angry at you. I've really had it. Go pick on someone else!"

You know you have your choices. You can go through life as an angry, bitter, cynical person or you have a choice to try to resolve it whatever way is best for you. If it is not a belief in God, you have to resolve it some other way.

Bob: I think you are going to be measured in life some way. You're given a problem and how did you handle it? You know. And then you have to make the best of it.

D.L.: Where were your supports?

Bob: Well, we had each other and we got a lot of support from our families. We also got a lot of support from our kids with Andrew's accident.

D.L.: How do you think Andrew was affected by having two deaf siblings?

Susan: He used to say things like "Poor me. I'm in the middle between two deaf kids and now I've got learning disabilities." He was always very manipulative.

Bob: Always when a crisis would arise, he was like an only child. He had no one to sit and talk to. The other two would get together and talk with each other, and he would be like the odd man out.

Susan: Andrew had to do the sharing with the others, but there was never any camaraderie among them.

Bob: The give and take. He would try to do it, but it just didn't work out. I don't think he would even bring his friends around.

D.L.: Was Andrew left out?

Susan: He wasn't left out. He sort of put himself out, I think.

Bob: Andrew got more attention than the other two, I would say. It was mainly his sports I got involved with. I tried to coach everything he was involved with. I think a lot of that was because he was between the other two. We spent a lot of time with him. I think, in spite of everything, he is going to turn out to be a nice adult.

Susan: Sometimes it's just in the kids. You can try and give them a good example and try and help them make proper decisions, do certain things, and sometimes kids are just not going to do things. That's why I don't take the credit for how well Timothy and Nancy are turning out and I don't take the blame for Andrew.

Bob: You look at the other two. Well, we did something right there. They are such nice human beings. And Andrew just chose a different road and it just caught up with him. I had warned him that he was traveling in the fast lane. Emotionally, the last few years, we have been so involved with him, almost to the detriment of the others. I sometimes get mad about that.

Susan: We feel that with this accident he has gotten a second chance. That's the way we are handling it with him. 'We don't understand why these things happen. Your best friend has died in the accident and you've been badly hurt. You are being given a second chance.'' And he seems to be changing. Nobody ever is the same after a head injury. But he's now giving talks to other kids about drugs. I always knew he experimented with drugs, but I had no idea he was so involved. He was very crafty about hiding it. Now he goes regularly to the rehabilitation program.

It's just one more thing and it's a big one. You just have to take it one day at a time.

D.L.: Are you coping with this better because of your experience with the deafness?

Susan: I'm sure that that has helped. People were also very supportive, our family especially.

D.L.: Do you see any good coming out of this?

Susan: I think it sort of sets your priorities. I think our values would be different if we didn't have these kids. I guess you could also say how you've grown in some areas. But who needed this?

Bob: You know you have taken a very difficult problem and coped with it, so that makes you feel pretty good about yourself. A lot of people admire us and that makes you feel good.

Susan: I've always maintained that you don't really have too many choices.

Bob: Exactly. You could jump out the window if you wanted to, but that's not going to solve any problems. You just have to hang in there.

Susan: It's been hard but all three kids are turning out okay. You have to sort of look at life as a journey that you go through, and it's how you wind up in the end.

D.L.: And you think you are winding up okay?

Susan: Yes, so far!

The Marshalls are a testament to the strength and resiliency in all of us, which we do not know we possess until we are tested. And they are being tested in full measure. The primary supports for Susan are her husband and her belief in God. Having a tragedy in one's life always causes a reevaluation of one's religious beliefs in the broadest sense of the word, and people must somehow reconcile the notion of a beneficent God with the awful events happening to them. Parents very often feel that either God is wicked for having done this to them or that they were wicked in some way that God needed to punish them. Susan has solved this dilemma by choosing to believe that God gave her these children to test her and she will be rewarded in an afterlife. Her belief system also permits her to be very angry at God; her God is a very personal one that she can address at will, and this enables her to maintain her own emotional homeostasis.

An existential crisis always surrounds the search for meaning in tragic occurrences, and professionals need to allow the family members the scope to search for meaning without imposing their own views. Some families adopt conventional religious explanations, while others have unique explanations for the tragedy that has occurred. How a family responds is variable. In a parent group, a mother commented, "Since this happened [deafness in her child], I have not been to attend church." Another mother in the group responded, "Since this happened I've been to church every Sunday."

As Gallagher, Cross, and Scharfman (1981) found, the families successful in coping with having a handicapped child were those in which there was a strong parental bond, high maternal self-esteem, and a strong set of supporting values; e.g., religion. Venters (1981) found that families who were successful in coping with the problem of cystic fibrosis in their children needed to make philosophic sense of the disease in order to cope with it. In the broadest sense of the term, there is always a religious crisis surrounding the birth of a deaf child, and Susan found in her religious views a strong support for coping with three handicapped children. I think this family would be judged as quite successful.

Successfully coping does not mean that, at times, the parent is not overwhelmed with grief and in need of help from others. Parents do not always see this. The grief process is a long one and it tends to go in cycles, with periods of seeming calm and acceptance then periods of grief, depression, and helplessness. One can be a strong person and cry, and occasionally have to ask for help. Very often family members do not seek help or feel guilty about their tears, because they would be seen as weak. Paradoxically, only the truly strong are willing to allow other people to witness their pain and helplessness.

I think what Susan calls depression is really grief at the losses in her life. Andrew was the only so-called normal child in the family; now, she and Bob realize that he is their most handicapped child. They both have lost the dream of being parents of a normal child. This is a terrible loss for all parents. In this case, it is more so because he was the only one of their three children who was normal.

It is tempting to blame Andrew's drug and alcohol dependency on his family position. However, many youngsters have a similar problem without having deaf siblings, and it is problematical whether he would be in similar difficulties with hearing siblings. Certainly, his parents were aware of his precarious family position, and they made every effort to compensate for his being an "outsider." It is very difficult for the Marshalls to not feel some guilt about Andrew's accident and drug abuse, but at some point, parents must acknowledge that they have done the best they knew how to do and coping with life is now the child's responsibility. I think the Marshalls are coming to this realization with all of their children.

Nancy Marshall's view:

Growing up in a hearing world is a great challenge for a person with a hearing loss, like me. There were times of difficulties and unhappiness.

I had a joyous childhood, with many friends from public school and in the neighborhood. I also have nice family relationships with my parents, two brothers, and many other relatives who love me. Although I was quiet as a child, I had no problem making friends. However, when my high school years approached, socializing started to become a demanding problem for me. It was part of adolescent years when teens worry about their own behavior and reactions toward others, especially in a group. There are times that people don't understand me, nor I, them. It takes time and courage to make strong friends with others, but a lot of people don't have that patience. As a result, I didn't, and still don't, totally fit well with either the hearing people or deaf people who use sign language as their major communication. I am trying to pick up sign language now.

I believe a beneficial way for persons with handcaps to improve their social life is to try to get involve [sic] in extracurricular activities and organizations and make an effort to be more outgoing. That is what I did in high school, and I made a few friends and it improved my self-esteem. It was tough for me to get through this and it was not always easy. However, there are times that I wish there are more people who have the same problems like me. It's good to have friends with the same handicap. These kind of friendships share the same feelings and can comfort each other about their problems. That's what I feel toward my younger brother, who is also hearing impaired. All the years we have been growing up, we have had a lot of conversations about our dilemmas in school, at home, and in social gatherings. We also have solved our problems trying to accept the fact that we are not the only ones with problems and there are people in this world that are worse off than one of us. We're really comfortable and understand each other, and sometimes we just laugh our problems off.

I'm proud to be getting an excellent education with help from teachers and some students. I also get a lot of language and learning skills from my mother, ever since I was small. I would not be what I am today without them. Being with the hearing people has made me make the effort to speak accurately, which is crucial for communication in a hearing society. Also, being with hearing people presents a great challenge for them to learn about deafness. I am always fortunate to help others acquire knowledge about how deaf people function in a hearing society, such as communication through sign language and TTY, close caption decoders, and other devices and services that improve the lives of the hearing impaired. It is something that hearing individuals don't have nor understand, just like the things that people with hearing loss can't do or have difficulty with in the hearing world. This sometimes has made me feel that I am not only handicapped toward others, but them towards me. I really appreciate the fact there are people who are cognizant about our problems and are trying to their best to provide in a hearing world. Our society has come a long way towards awareness of deafness and providing more services for them since Alexander Graham Bell's time.

Nancy Marshall

Timothy Marshall's view:

Some days I think about being deaf and other times I don't think about it. I have an older brother and sister, and I get a lot of advice from them. Being the youngest is great because I have my brother and sister.

My high school is a good school, because there are good teachers and also I have a good basketball coach, which I am comfortable with. I keep busy with X-C, basketball, track. Being a teenager is tough and sometimes I feel I'm missing a lot with hearing kids. If I was with a group of deaf kids, it would be easier that [sic] with the hearing kids.

Timothy Marshall

REFERENCES

Gallagher, J. J., Cross, A., & Scharfman, W. (1981). Parental adaptation to a young handicapped child: The father's role. *Journal of the Division for Early Childhood, 3*, 3-14.

Venters, M. (1981). Familial coping with chronic and severe childhood illness: The case of cystic fibrosis. *Social Science and Medicine, 15A*, 289–297.

CHAPTER 7

Grandparents

Grandparenthood is the ultimate developmental phase of parenthood. It is the opportunity to reap a second harvest; within our culture, it is the "childless parenthood" phase of the life cycle. As one grandparent put it, "One can have all the fun of being a parent and none of the responsibility."

In some cultures, the grandparents have minimal roles and responsibilities and, at times, are considered superfluous, as in crises such as food shortages. One can easily conjure visions of the Eskimo grandparent sitting on an ice floe waiting to die from exposure, because he or she is no longer useful to the community.

In other cultures, grandparents are considered the heads of the extended clan and are ancillary parents with an available fount of experience, which is drawn upon when some predicament overtakes the family. In the Maori culture, grandparents have primary responsibility for child rearing. The parents will work in the fields while the grandparents stay home to raise the child. There is an assumption within the culture that it takes maturity and wisdom to raise children, which only the grandparents possess. As a soon-to-be grandfather, I often think of the Maori system of child rearing and I am not sure it would work for me. I think much of my current wisdom in parenting has come from going through the experience and making mistakes. Whatever child-rearing wisdom I possess is hard won and fully earned. At this point, I prefer the role of a very interested consultant and I will leave the parenting responsibilities to my children.

Currently, in the United States, 70 percent of persons over age 65 are grandparents and a sizeable number of persons age 55–65 also are grandparents (Kivnick, 1982). The grandparent, however, seems to be rapidly disappearing as an active family member. Kornhaber and Woodward (1985) report on interviews of 300 grandparents and grandchildren. They found that only 15 percent of the families included an actively involved grandparent. The majority (70 percent) were intermittently involved, and 15 percent of the grandparents were not involved at all. They feel that a new social contract is in effect, which allows the parents to define the grandparents' role, and that the new role diminishes grandparent involvement.

Based on the in-depth interviews of the children, they found that families benefitted from closely connected grandparents. Grandparents functioned as mentors, caretakers, mediators between child and parents, same-sex role models, and family historians. Grandparents were also compeling, valuable models for old age; they stimulated the children to anticipate their own aging and death without fear, and children with actively involved grandparents were able to generalize their feelings to other older people. From this study, there does not seem to be any negative effects of grandparent involvement; however, parent were not interviewed and there may very well be increased stress in families with active grandparents.

The grandparent is able to offer the child a pure, simple, unselfish emotional attachment that remains stable throughout the child's life. The relationship with the parents, while always the primary relationship, is inherently unstable as the child grows into adulthood. As a young adult once remarked, "I always knew that even if the police were on my tail and I had committed the most heinous crime that my grandparents would take me in." A cynic has also commented that grandparents and grandchildren have a deep relationship because they share a common enemy. Kornhaber and Woodward conclude that the connection between grandparent and grandchild is natural and second in emotional power only to the primordial bond between parent and child, "and that a caring grandparent can be a great parent forever— as long as the vital connection is established early in the child's life." As one might expect, the authors also found that the grandchildren had a very positive effect on the grandparent; actively connected grandparents were much happier and more vital than uninvolved grandparents.

The influence of grandparents extends beyond the early childhood experiences. Hartshorne and Manaster (1982) studied the relationship of grandparents to young adults (age 21). They interviewed and tested 178 college students and found that their grandparents' relationship was still very important to the grandchildren. Ninety percent of the subjects wished they had more contact with their grandparents than they currently do and 95 percent of the grandchildren rated the importance of their relationship with their grandparents as either extremely important (44 percent) or important (51 percent). The grandparent that consistently received the highest rating of importance was the mother's mother. In many families apparently there is a great deal of bonding between the mother's mother and the grandchild. Kahana and Kahana (1970) also found that the maternal grandmother was the most important grandparent. It is clear that grandparents can be very important individuals to the grandchild, yet we still do not have very much experimental evidence as to just what their influence is.

Even when remote, grandparents are "present" in every family. We always carry our family of origin into our new nuclear family. Our images of what constitutes marriage and parenthood stems from our childhood experiences, where we observe and assess our parents' parenting and our parents' marriage. We carry that image with us when we start our new family, either by imitating our parents or by being determined to do the opposite: in short, being our antiparent. In either case, we are influenced by them. Only with time and thought can we begin to find our own way into marital and parenting roles based on our own direct experiences. Some of the change comes about in initial phases of family formation due to the stress of melding the spouses' disparate personal paradigms into the family paradigm. Our ideas of the "appropriate normal" stem from our families of origin. We always are amazed to find that our spouse has a different appropriate normal and we must negotiate in order to develop an appropriate normal for the newly formed family.

Ironically, another point at which parents can reevaluate their marriage and their parenting is when they have a handicapped child. The stress of the deafness will very often cause a reexamination of the role structure formed by the parents from their experiences in their own families of origin. Programs and professionals need to be sensitive to the reevaluation process that parents undergo. This is a very fertile time for positive change in the family paradigm.

There do not appear to be any studies on the influence of grandparents in families with a deaf child, despite the acknowledgment by almost everyone who has written in the field that grandparents play an enormously important role. I suspect this results from the huge variability in the grandparents' roles in the nuclear family. In some families, grandparents are deceased or live far away; sometimes grandparents live near the family but are psychologically remote. In other families, grandparents play a very active role and may live with the family or be physically or psychologically very close. The extreme variability of the grandparents' roles confounds most research designs.

Grandparents are seldom neutral factors in the life of a family with a handicapped child. They can be tremendously supportive, as Poppa in the Wagner family, who fulfilled many of the parental functions with the hearing siblings and allowed the parents to focus on the deafness. Bill Wagner's father took on the chore of driving once a week to bring Laura home from school. He also came to the home and was emotionally supportive the first week that Laura was enrolled in the school for the deaf. Both the Wagner and Marshall grandparents were the first to diagnose the deafness. On the other hand, grandparents can be very draining, as were the grandparents in the Murphy family, who in the early years never got beyond feeling sorry for Robert and seemed to require more support from their children than they could give.

Harris, Handelman, and Palmer (1985), by way of a questionnaire, interviewed the mothers, fathers, grandmothers, and grandfathers of 19 autistic children. They found that the grandparents had a consistently more optimistic view of the child's limitations than the parents. They also noted that grandparents tended to deny the child's handicap long after it had been accepted by the parents. They, too, found that the most familial support was provided by the maternal grandmother. The importance of the maternal grandparent as a support to the family was also found by Gath (1978) in her study of families with a Down's syndrome child and is quite consistent with the findings of studies of normal families.

There are several nonempirical discussions in the literature of the grandparents' role in a handicapped family. For example, Berns (1980) points out the potentially useful role that grandparents can have in supporting the parents and giving the handicapped child a sense of value. McPhee (1982) is a maternal grandmother, who poignantly describes how she came to love and accept her cerebral palsied grandson.

One event that does occur in many families with a deaf child is an exacerbation of the normal life-cycle crisis when the parents realize that they know more than their parents and experience an existential loneliness. Having a deaf child almost invariably shortens the time span for the crisis. Shortly after they learn that they have a deaf child, parents frequently seek support and guidance from their own parents. Often, they discover that they know far more about deafness than their own parents and a role reversal occurs, much as Mrs. Murphy noted, whereby the parents comfort, guide, and inform the grandparents.

Conversely, the crisis of the deafness is very often the first time that the grandparents realize that their child is now an adult. The role reversal usually occurs much sooner than the parents or grandparents are prepared for. Parents very often feel cheated because they are not getting the support they need. Grandparents are very often scared, confused, and suffering a double grief because, not only is their grandchild "hurting," their own child is grieving, too. I think the predominant feeling of most grandparents at this time is one of helplessness, which makes it very hard for them to offer support.

It is not uncommon for grandparents to be locked into denial, sure that the child will "outgrow" the deafness or that "they" will find a cure for it. They keep trying to reassure the parents of this; and the parents, who are better informed and have emotionally accepted the child's deafness, find that relating to the grandparents drains their own emotional resources. They are constantly forced to provide support for their parents when they are hard pressed to maintain their own emotional stability. Neither Lydia Wagner or Jean Murphy felt that she could share her feelings with her parents.

On the other hand, grandparents can be both emotionally supportive, and provide much needed help to the family by providing childcare or fulfilling some of the neglected parental functions with the hearing siblings. They also can be emotionally supportive, as they apparently were in the Marshall family.

Grandparents' feelings parallel very closely the parents' responses. They feel grief, anger, anxiety, and guilt in varying proportions. They display their feelings to their children and to professionals in accordance with the cultural values of their family. More often than not, there is no openness about feelings between grandparents and parents. Very frequently, neither one wants to burden the other with their pain; they are very protective of each other. Unfortunately, this can be misinterpreted as indifference, and grandparents can be viewed as cold and uninvolved; when, in reality, they are frightened and concerned but very diffident about sharing their feelings. The parents and grandparents often need help in bridging the gap between them. Pieper (1976) makes an eloquent plea for general understanding between parent and grandparent, noting how much support they can give each other, and she calls for open discussion groups between parents and grandparents to enhance and develop that support.

A technique I have used frequently with good success in workshops containing parents and grandparents is known as the *fish bowl design*. In this procedure, the grandparents first sit in a circle to discuss what it is like to be the grandparent of a deaf child, while the parents sit on the periphery. (Only people sitting in the center group may talk and no one is required to talk.) After a while, the parents and grandparents exchange seats, with the parents discussing what it is like to be a parent of a deaf child. When the parents have finished, the whole group joins together to share what they have learned. The fish bowl design forces the outer group to listen, while the people in the center know that there are eavesdroppers. The group process usually fosters an openness that is not present in some families. This design also permits cross-familial learning; that is, the sharing of experiences among different families. It is much easier to "hear" a parent or grandparent speak, when that person is not a relative. Defensiveness is not present and the need to protect from pain also is not there. Groups such as this almost invariably spark a great deal of family dialogue. They also are the most professionally satisfying groups that I lead.

Some families are very open with their feelings, and there is a free exchange of affect between the parents and grandparents. In other families, there is a minimum of openness and feelings are very well hidden, or are expressed very minimally and would be missed by most outside observers. Each family has its own way of dealing with crises and there is nothing unique to the crises generated by having a deaf child. The family paradigm for dealing with all crises will emerge in the course of coping with the particular crisis caused by the child's deafness. Let's listen to some grandparents.

These were going to be our best years. My husband retired and we moved near our daughter. When we found out that our grandson was deaf, it was like the roof fell in. For the first three months, we used to wake up each morning and cry. There has never been anything like this in our family, ever. For the first few months, we could not even talk with our daughter. She was so sharp with me. There was so much anger. Now, it is better and she talks with me, but we are afraid that they are going to move to be near the school for the deaf and we will lose them again.

I never could talk to my son about our grandaughter's deafness. He would always shut me out, even when he was a little boy. And now, I know he is hurting and I can't talk with him.

Our grandaughter's deafness has brought us together. My daughter has grown up so much in having to take care of this child. Frankly, I didn't think she could do it. She was always so immature. I really admire her now. She is a responsible woman, who is coping very well with a very difficult problem.

I feel so helpless I don't know what to do. All I seem able to do these days is to say "poor me," "my poor children" and "my poor grandchild" and I know that that is not helpful.

It is very frustrating to me to be so far away. I don't really know what is going on. Getting information on the phone is very unsatisfactory. I am confident my daughter can do this. She is very capable. I wish I could help her more.

At this point in time, we know almost nothing about grandparents. They appear to be a badly underresearched, underutilized resource to the family.

REFERENCES

Berns, J. (1980). Grandparents of handicapped children. *Social Work, 25,* 238–239.

Gath, A. (1978). *Down's syndrome and the family—The early years.* London: Academic Press.

Harris, S., Handlman, J., & Palmer, C. (1985). Parents and grandparents view the autistic child. *Journal of Autism and Developmental Disorders, 15,* (2), 125–135.

Hartshorne, T., & Manaster, G. (1982). The relationship with grandparents: Contact, importance, role conception. *International Aging and Human Development, 15,* (3), 233–244.

Kahana, B., & Kahana, E. (1970). Children's views of their grandparents: Influences of the kinship system. *The Gerontologist, 10,* 39–44.

Kivnick, H. (1982). Grandparenthood: An overview of meaning and mental health. *The Gerontologist, 22,* 59–66.

Kornhaber, C. and Woodward, L. (1985). *Grandparents/Grandchildren—The vital connection.* New Brunswick, NJ: Transaction Books.

McPhee, N. (1982). A very special magic—A grandmother's delight. *The Exceptional Parent, 12,* 13–16.

Pieper, E. (1976). Grandparents can help. *The Exceptional Parent, 6,* 7–9.

CHAPTER 8

Working with the Deaf Family

In some respects, the title of this chapter is inaccurate,the deafness is characteristic of only one family member. Yet, the title reflects the theme of the book, that the deafness affects everyone in the family and, in reality, one is dealing with a "deaf family." In order to be most effective in ameliorating the effects of deafness on the family, the professional must always keep in mind the notion of a family as a system in which all of the parts are intimately and inextricably linked; deafness in one member means that everyone in the family is to some degree deaf.

According to Minuchin, Rosman, and Baker (1978), two attributes of families are vital to its functioning: the nature of the family's boundaries and the capacity of the system to change in response to altered conditions.

BOUNDARIES

The extrafamilial boundaries, in effect, define the family from the rest of society. The family is formed first by the melding of the spouses' personal paradigms to form the family paradigm. As children are born or family members are added, such as the inclusion of a grandparent, intrafamilial boundaries are created. Thus, a growing family would have an executive subsystem that would be different than the enlarging sibling subsystem.

Every family subsystem has specific functions and, in order for a family to function effectively, there must be clarity in defining the limits and responsibilities of each subsystem and there must be freedom from undue interference in each system. For example, one of the primary functions of the sibling subsystem is to teach the children how to develop negotiation skills around conflicts and how to use these skills in their peer relationships. The parents must practice a kind of benign neglect to allow the siblings to resolve their own issues so they can learn these vital negotiating skills. Parents need to monitor the siblings' subsystem and mediate conflicts only when necessary.

CHANGE IN THE FAMILY

One of the family's most important tasks is to maintain continuity and stability in the face of a continuously changing reality. The need to belong (affiliation) is fundamental to our sense of well-being. The family provides the primary affiliation unit for the growing child. Yet, the family must deal with the disequilibrium inherent in the life cycle, as parents age and children move rapidly through the developmental stages. Eventually, the growth of the children must be met with change in the organization of the family. Authority must continuously be ceded by the parents, until ultimately they have none. At some point, parents must face the implications of their child's growth for their own sense of self: Energies that were formerly devoted to the parenting, now can be utilized within the marriage.

Change also comes from extrafamilial sources, such as job changes, family moves, or the inclusion of an aged grandparent within the family. Discovery of deafness in a child is a very powerful extrafamilial stress on the family system.

Stress on the family system per se is not bad. It is an impetus for growth and change, just as it is in the individual. Families must come to understand the sources of their stress and accommodate them. How the family responds to the change is a key element in the family structure. Almost all change is resisted at first because it is in conflict with the family's other primary function, to maintain stability. Within families, there is always a dynamic tension between the homeostatic forces and the elements of change. Change usually is accomplished most easily in small increments, which sometimes occur on a subconscious level; with the accumulation of the last critical increment, a paradigmatic shift can occur. Thus, parents gradually allow the child more responsibility without necessarily being very aware that they have been ceding their authority, until they suddenly become aware that their child is an adult. A parent once remarked, "I can remember my daughter as a 2 year old needing a great deal of supervision, and then it felt as if I slept late one morning and she was suddenly an adult."

Unfortunately, families and individuals do not always have the luxury of incremental change. Life exigencies sometimes force very rapid changes for which the family is not prepared. Deafness is one of those rapid changes forced on families.

THE DEAF FAMILY

Generally, deafness in a child interferes severely with the family's boundaries, forcing the family to make cataclysmic changes within a very short period of time. The extrafamilial boundary is pierced by professionals, who intrude into the family life. Suddenly, the audiologist and teacher of the deaf become "members" of the family. The information and advice, sometimes given so offhandedly, have profound effects on the family. And in some ways, the professionals become ancillary parents, sometimes inadvertently undermining the parents' authority.

When parents are informed that their child is deaf, they very often become quite tentative about exercising their parental authority. They become uncertain and insecure. Lydia Wagner, for example, felt that Laura's world was so unfamiliar to her that she did not know what her child's experiences were like. Parents also have a myth of the fragility of the deaf child; they feel that the child is so delicate that they cannot afford to make any mistakes, because to do so might damage the child irreparably. I am not sure of the origins of the myth, but I suspect in part it stems from the professionals' anxiety to move ahead rapidly without error and the parents' recognition of their own and their child's vulnerability. It takes considerable effort, by both parents and professionals, to reassert the executive authority that is so necessary to the maintenance of family stability and the child's emotional and social development.

It also is quite common for the deaf child to become the natural focus for whatever else goes wrong in the family, and he or she can very easily be triangulated into the parental system. One or both parents can develop an overclose relationship with the child, which excludes the other spouse and the other children. Usually, the mother excludes the father. In my clinical experience, this is more apt to happen in families in which the spouse system is weak to begin with and the mother/wife is getting little support or satisfaction from her husband. The child then can become a focus for the marital dissatisfaction.

The boundaries in the sibling subsystem also are frequently disturbed by the child's deafness. It is not uncommon for the oldest sister to assume many parental functions and for the younger siblings to have to assume responsibilities at an earlier age. Conflict and negotiation also are frequently distorted within the sibling system. Note, for example, Kate and Conrad's unwillingness to fight and tease Laura from both the point of view of her not understanding what was going on and the implicit injunction that permeated the family, that Laura was somehow more delicate than anyone else.

In addition to the boundary issue, the family must make the paradigmatic shift from being a normal family to being a deaf family. This is an enormous change that requires restructuring the roles for the entire family. Because the change generally is so frightening and seen at first as overwhelming, a denial mechanism is activated and the family resists any changes. Denial will manifest itself in several different ways. At the time of diagnosis, there often is some delay caused by the parents' unwillingness to confirm the possibility that the child may be deaf. There usually are problems with wearing the hearing aid: parents of newly diagnosed deaf children frequently discuss whether or not the child wears the hearing aid when a picture is taken; for families who have accepted the child's deafness, it is never an issue: the hearing aid is seen as a part of the child's anatomy.

The denial mechanism manifests itself throughout the course of raising the child. Anytime that the family is confronted with change, as, for example, to move the child from a mainstream program to a school for the deaf, as both Laura Wagner and Robert Murphy were, there will be a time lag until the family members adjust to the new reality. Anytime there is a threat to the family's homeostasis, resistence will be met.

The paradigmatic shift to a deaf family will occur when the family becomes convinced that (1) the family, especially the mother, has the resources and the power to make a difference and (2) the change will be in their and the child's best interest. In short, the family needs some hope and confidence that they can make a difference. At this point, professionals can be immensely helpful by providing the family with information, as needed, and by interacting with the family in such a way as to instill confidence in their ability to cope with the child's deafness.

SUCCESSFUL FAMILIES

One can glean from existing research that families judged to be successful in coping with a handicapped child seem to share certain characteristics (Gallagher, Cross, & Scharfman, 1981; Lavelle & Keogh, 1980; Longo & Bond, 1984; and Venters, 1981).

1 A feeling within the family that the burden is shared, both within and outside of the family. (I often tell parents that a successful deaf child is the result of the cooperation of thirds: one third parents, one third school, and one third child.)
2 The parents have a high degree of self-esteem and self-confidence.
3 The family has made philosophical sense of the situation.
4 Family members perceive that their behavior can make a difference.

In my experience, there are wide variations in how successful families function. Although the families have gone through some restructuring as a result of the deafness, the ultimate coping solution generally will be consistent with the original family paradigm. In families in which there is fairly traditional sex role definitions, with the mother having the primary child-rearing resonsibilities and the father having the primary economic responsibilities, the presence of a deaf child will exaggerate these roles, so that the mother will increase her child-rearing responsibilities, while the father will feel an exaggerated need to provide more economic means for the family. He knows, for example, that it is unlikely his wife will be able to work now that so much more of her energy will be devoted to the deaf child and that the financial demands on the family also will increase. Fathers frequently begin to work longer as a good excuse to leave the house and avoid their child or wife's grief, too. Work can become a convenient evasion of his familial responsibilities and of his guilt.

What generally is not appreciated by most professionals is that the father's role also is frequently restructured the most. He must become more suportive of his wife's efforts and must assume more of the child-rearing responsibility than he had previously. Very often, he is called upon to assume roles that are unfamiliar to him. In the Wagner family, Bill began building his business at the same time he recognized the need to support his wife and provide some relief for her: He gave lessons on Saturday mornings. Paul Murphy worked overtime a great deal to provide his wife the space to do the child rearing and, although he took no direct part in the child rearing, he was emotionally supportive of his wife. Bob Marshall also embarked on a heavy work load, yet found the time to became very much involved with Andrew's activities.

The family's unique style of adaptation must be respected by the professional. Families work in very different ways and professionals need to respect each coping strategy as long as the family remains functional. A coping strategy that requires an overinvolved mother may be necessary if the family is to turn out a successfully functioning deaf child. This solution will work if the mother feels that her burden is shared somewhat and she perceives that she has support, both within and outside of her family.

Very often, women professionals, who are at a different state of social consciousness than the children's mothers, tend to judge a family as deficient when it is run along traditional sex role stereotypes. These families are sometimes quite successful and quite functional; the family must not be judged but accepted. Families always must be accepted for what they are rather than for what the professional feels they should be.

I think the ultimately successful family is able to get the deafness in perspective and learns to enjoy the youngster as a child who happens not to hear too well. There are many routes to accomplish this. The professional must learn to respect the boundaries of the family and try to repair those boundaries damaged by the deafness by always working to enhance the self-esteem of the family members; one must always be seeking to empower families.

One must always keep in mind that we professionals are usually dealing with functional families that, by virtue of our interventions, we are trying to make more optimal; dysfunctional families need to be referred for family therapy. Increasingly, the literature recognizes the need for family therapists to concern themselves with the problems of the deaf family; and, it is hoped, that many communities will be able to offer family therapy to the dysfunctional deaf family (Harvey, 1984; Mendelsohn & Rozek, 1983; Robinson & Weathers, 1974; and Shapiro & Harris, 1976).

PROFESSIONAL INTERVENTIONS

Currently, research indicates that intervention by professionals' is not always helpful. Sandow and Clarke (1977) studied the effects of a home intervention program on the performance of severely subnormal preschool children, mainly those with Down's syndrome and severe cerebral palsy. The 32 children were divided into two matched groups. In a three-year study, one group of families was visited by a therapist once every two weeks for a two-hour session, while the other group was visited once every two months. The children were periodically tested for progress on their cognitive functioning and speech and language development. The findings were rather startling. Initially, the more frequently visited children showed more gains in intellectual growth and in speech and language than the less frequently visited children. As the study progressed, however, the researchers found that the less frequently visited children showed a greater rise in performance after the initial decrement than the more frequently visited children. This gain increased into the third year of the study. The researchers interpret their data to suggest that parents in the less frequently visited group were less dependent on the visiting therapist and more able to take positive action in assisting their children and improving their situation than the more frequently visited parents.

The Sandow and Clarke study agrees with my own impression from observing groups of itinerant teachers who tend to take over the therapy, fostered by their eagerness to demonstrate their own competency and their anxiety to do things well. (This finding is not restricted to itinerant teachers; clinic-based teachers/therapists exhibit the same behaviors.) To ensure that the child gets a good lesson, the teacher takes control of the child and the therapy, undermining the parents' confidence. When the teacher has only a very limited time to see a family, there is a strong desire to ensure success, and the teacher tends to give the lesson with the mother observing. These lessons are usually successful because the child has a limited, positive contact with the teacher and, one can assume, the teacher is competent. The teacher then tells the parent to continue working on this lesson during the intervening week. When the parent tries to follow through on what has been demonstrated, she invariably fails. The failure occurs for a variety of reasons. The child is too familiar with the parent and resents the parent as a teacher. The parent is too emotionally involved with the child and is not able to see the child clearly. Finally, there is no reason to assume that the parent is very competent in giving lessons: Why should he or she be? In programs where the professionals consistently demonstrate their competence, the parents' confidence is undermined subtly. In fact, the parents are subtly programmed to fail. Lowering the parents' self-confidence tends to foster parental dependency.

Professionals need to learn that, in many situations, the most helpful strategy is to not help or, at least, to help in a covert way. Very often not doing is as important as doing and clinical wisdom requires knowing when to act. My own bias about itinerant programs is that they should be almost entirely parent-centered and that the teacher should interact minimally with the child. The parent should do most of the lesson and the teacher should focus on those things that the parent is doing well, so as to bolster confidence. I think professionals are much more helpful when their assistance is not apparent than when the families exclaim, "What would we ever do without you!" The latter families invariably remain dependent and, in the long term, may produce children who do not progress very far because they lack effective parents. We cannot have a "savior" without some loss of self-esteem.

Another way professionals can help families function better is by teaching them to be more direct in their communication. This helps them to find strategies for resolving conflict and for expressing their caring for one another. Communication in families needs to be direct, with ownership of feelings. The principal mechanism for accomplishing better communication within the family is by modeling the optimal behaviors for the family members. In one sense of the word, for a time, the professional parents the parents and, as in any good parenting process, helps to create independent, well-functioning adults who no longer need them.

The Diagnostic Process

The diagnostic process demonstrated to me during my training as a clinical audiologist, and that I followed during the first years of my professional life, consisted of taking a case history, then trying to separate the child from the parents, and afterwards "counseling" the parents. In the counseling, I attempted to explain my test procedures and the results of the tests. I have come to see that this is not a very effective clinical procedure; among other things, the parent is not able to deal with much cognitive material at this point. There is experimental support for this point of view. Williams and Darbyshire (1982) interviewed 25 families within a year of the child's diagnosis of deafness. Eighty-four percent of the families felt that most parents are not able to understand all the information they are given by audiologists. Moreover, when asked to restate the audiologist's explanation of what hearing loss would mean to their child, 40 percent of the families could not give any answer, and a further 24 percent answered in a way that the examiners felt was incorrect. In total,

64 percent of the families left the audiological testing without a clear idea of their child's handicap and its implications to them.

I have found, over the years, that one cannot go any faster than the parent is willing or able to go. Audiologists, I think, limit truly effective case management when they become so overwhelmed by their own anxiety to get a hearing aid on the child and to get the child into an educational program that they try to bypass the parents grief and "slowness" in acquiring information through a very active management of the case or by inundating the parents with a great deal of information. This invariably leads to passive, dependent parents and to ineffective management in the long run.

The way in which audiological examinations are conducted can also contribute to the parents' difficulty in accepting the deafness and in acquiring information. When the parents cannot actually see their child's deafness objectified, they can fantasize that perhaps there was some mistake, that the audiologist or the equipment might have failed in some way, so as to give an erroneous result. (Most people have mixed feelings about technology. Machines generally are believed to be infallible but events, such as the recent space shuttle disaster and the Russian nuclear plant explosion, point out that machines and the people who run them are quite fallible.) It becomes hard for the parents to accept the "death" of their child's hearing much as it is hard for the families of Vietnam veterans missing in action to accept their deaths when no corpse has been found.

Denial is fostered whenever there is a separation of the person from the event. There is a great deal of folk wisdom, for example, in the traditional funeral service, in which the grieving family goes to the chapel and views the corpse then follows the hearse to the cemetery and watches the coffin lowered into the ground. This is immensely painful for the family but psychologically very sound. The family cannot deny the death, and they must then begin the painful process of accommodating the loss.

When I told parents who had not viewed the testing that their child could not hear, they were very often hostile. The hostility was based on fear but I did not always see that. People very frequently "kill" the messenger when they don't like the message. This diagnostic strategy also set me up as the expert and the parents as the passive recipients of my expertise and information, a clinical dynamic that is destructive to the goal of creating self-confident, empowered families.

The diagnostic process I have evolved involves the whole family in determining the child's hearing status. Initially, I take a minimal case history from the family. I am most interested in finding out their expectations from the examination, then I enlist them as codiagnosticians with me in the task of determining the child's hearing. All family members are urged to come into the test room with me, this includes any siblings or grandparents who accompany the parents. Together, we form the diagnostic team and I explain the procedures I employ. I usually have one family member fill in the audiogram as together we determine the child's hearing status. If we cannot agree on the child's response to a sound, we test again. Time and time again, I have been struck at how immensely creative families have been in evolving techniques for testing the child's hearing. This has been especially true of older siblings, who very often take over the task of conditioning the child to the sound stimuli.

After we have determined that the child is hearing impaired, I do not give the family much information. At this point, they usually are pretty overwrought and cannot process much information. One mother commented that "When I realized that my child was deaf, all I wanted to do was go someplace and hide." I usually ask them "What do you need to know?" and answer any questions that emerge. I do not answer in any great detail. People generally are ready for information when they can start articulating questions on their own. I also will ask them how they are feeling; usually I get a response such as "numb," since the family members are in a state of shock. I usually give the family the name and phone number of parents of older deaf children who have agreed to talk with parents of newly diagnosed children. The family seldom calls, as the denial mechanism is still operative. (I don't think any clinical procedure can avoid or completely eliminate denial. Denial is the last defense against complete psychological devastation and, as such, it is very necessary.)

On subsequent visits, more information is gradually given and more feelings begin to emerge. When they have reminisced with me about the diagnostic process, parents have recalled the pain of sitting in a room, listening to the sounds come through the speaker and seeing their child not respond. They also have commented how glad they were that I was there with them as they went through the ordeal.

Listening

Professionals are expected to perform. This expectation is fostered in the training program where listening is not seen as an active clinical procedure. There is a pervasive expectation that the professional's job is to inform and advise; families also expect this from professionals. Yet, I think there is no more powerful intervention for a professional than to listen responsively to the family.

Listening is a highly validating behavior. It says to the client, "What you have to say is important to me; I want to spend time getting to know you and to understand how the world looks to you." Listening also conveys that the individual possesses some wisdom, has something of value to say. Through the careful listening, a professional helps the family reveal its paradigm and coping mechanisms. Listening also is the basic mechanism for the establishment of trust.

Good listening is not the appearance of listening, where the professional is silent but is thinking of the next response or trying to find some weakness in the clients' arguments, so as to persuade them. In order to be a good listener, one must not have a point of view. One needs to be caring, responsive, and nonjudgmental.

Careful responsive listening allows the release of the pent-up emotions that most parents hold within themselves and that can be quite destructive. When the clinician is caring, responsive, and, above all, nonjudgmental; when the clinician's attitude acknowledges that feelings just *are*, not right or wrong but just the way the parents feel; then the parents can more readily take constructive action, free of immobilization from unacknowledged feelings. LeMaistre (1985), a psychologist who has multiple sclerosis, wrote movingly about people with chronic illness. She states,

> In the face of such losses to experience fear, anger, depression and anxiety is normal. . . . serious emotional difficulties are more often the lot of people who do not acknowledge the emotional stress they feel and thereby bottle up depression or anxiety until these feelings are so powerful they break through their defenses. By the time an emotion has become this powerful, it is much more difficult to survive its impact without severe scarring (p. 17).

Chinn, Winn, and Walters (1978) wrote extensively about the role of responsive listening in communication with parents of children who have special needs. For them, responsive listening (1) is empathic, (2) labels specific feelings not general ones, (3) begins by focusing on current feelings, and (4) assures that the listener's nonverbal messages are congruent with those expressed verbally. In responsive listening, the receiver sends back an empathic message that indicates that the hearer not only understood the words but the underlying feelings as well. The listening is a component of a relationship that reflects deep respect, acceptance, and warmth. For examples of reflective listening, the reader is urged to examine again the family interviews in this book.

Careful, responsive listening in the clinical interaction stimulates marvelous growth. An anonymously written poem that I found recently says it all.

LISTEN
When I ask you to listen to me
and you start giving advice
you have not done what I asked.

When I ask you to listen to me
and you begin to tell me why I shouldn't
feel that way,
you are trampling on my feelings.

When I ask you to listen to me
and you feel you have to do something to
solve my problem,
you have failed me, strange as that may
seem.

Listen! All I asked, was that you listen.
not talk or do—just hear me.
Advice is cheap: 10 cents will get you both
Dear Abbey and Billy Graham in the same
newspaper.

And I can do for myself; I'm not helpless.
Maybe discouraged and faltering, but not
helpless.

When you do something for me that I can and
need to do for myself, you contribute to
my fear and weakness.

But, when you accept as a simple fact that I do
feel what I feel, no matter how
irrational, then I can get about the
business of understanding what's
behind this irrational feeling.
And when that's clear, the answers are
obvious and I don't need advice.

Irrational feelings make sense when we
understand what's behind them.

Perhaps that's why prayer works, sometimes, for
some people, because God is mute, and He

doesn't give advice or try to fix things.
"They" just listen and let you work it out
for yourself.

So, please listen and just hear me. And, if
you want to to talk, wait a minute for
your turn; and, I'll listen to you.

Anonymous

Enhancing Self-Esteem

All clinical procedures followed with families need to be evaluated in terms of whether they enhance the self-esteem of the family members. Generally, the most self-enhancing procedures are those in which family members actively participate and can experience some success. When there is some success, families come to trust their own capabilities. As Featherstone (1980) so eloquently put it, "Fears ease as experience discredits fantasy, as mothers and fathers learn that actual problems of raising their child differ from the ones they imagined. Similarly, small victories over private demons reassure parents about their own ability to raise their child" (p. 27).

Professionals need to realize that they can be more helpful by working in a much less overt way. Professionals need to take the point of view that parents will make good decisions about their children, albeit with some mistakes. The communication of this quiet confidence to parents enhances their self-esteem. The professional who cannot develop such confidence in the parents should not work with the family. In a healthy clinical relationship, the parent and clinician are coequals. Understanding and collaboration are essential. Each learns from the other and together they arrive at new insights.

Building confidence requires a much more active parental role than is seen in most schools and clinics. A confident mother of a deaf child put it well when she said, "When we first learned that Michael was deaf, everyone told us what to do and we listened; now we question."

Therapists need to set up situations whereby the parents can experience some success in working with their children, especially in the early stages of the parent-professional interaction. Unfortunately, ours is often seen as a deficit profession; we seek to remediate. We start looking at the things that the child, the parent, and the professional are not doing right, to institute corrective procedures. This is not the best way to look at people who are learning new skills; it is far better to focus on what the child and parent are doing right and move from there. By focusing on the pluses in the situation, the deficits disappear. It all becomes a matter of how a professional chooses to look at the clinical/learning process. An affirming, positive view enhances self-esteem. It allows people to risk and encourages growth. Beginning with a deficit model enhances deficiencies, which lowers self-esteem, reduces willingness to risk, and encourages dependency.

The model I prefer for teachers interacting with a family in the initial stages involves first asking the parents what they thought their child needed and what they thought would work best with their child. The parents need to be enlisted as coteachers who have something of value to give. Most parents approach those intitial situations as though they have nothing to offer and all wisdom and power reside with the teacher. Unfortunately, too many teachers feel that way, too. The teacher then needs to allow the parent to interact with the child. Teachers should start by asking the parent what worked well during the therapy. Parents often need help seeing what went well, as they also often view learning as a remediative process. At all times, the professionals must work to maintain a locus of control within the parents, so that the parents determine the extent and pace of their own learning.

Teachers can help insecure parents most by limiting the initial therapeutic tasks, so that both the parents and the child experience some success early in the process; sometimes, and for some parents, the task needs to be as simple as getting the ear mold inserted. At all stages, parents are asked what they need to know and what they think they are ready to learn next. When parents are self-confident and secure, the teacher can begin to actively work with the child as a demonstration of things to be done.

Reframing

A technique of changing a deficit perception to an affirmative one is known as *reframing*. It helps a person look at the "problem" from a different perspective; for example, the problem becomes challenge. External events have no meaning until we give meaning to them. Our glass can either be half full or half empty, depending on how we choose to view it. The teacher, either by modeling a reframing comment or by gently redirecting the family member's comment, can change a family's perception and, therefore, its behavior. For example,

Comment: There are so few programs for me to choose for my child.

Reframing: It seems like you now have a chance to start a needed program.

Comment: I am tired of strangers' questions.

Reframing: What a nice opportunity to educate someone.

Comment: Why me?

Reframing: Why not you?

Comment: Who asked for this?

Reframing: Yours is now an especially interesting life.

Reframing must be done very sensitively; the timing and intonation must be exquisite. If it is not, the professional might be seen as an insensitive clod or a Pollyanna who just doesn't understand the problem. Reframing is best left to the latter stages of the grief process, when the family is ready to move on to constructive action. All successful families must somehow find meaning and direction in the child's deafness. I think the ultimate goal of working with families is to help the parents make something positive happen as a result of having a hearing-impaired child. Probably, the ultimate reframing question asked of family members is How can you make this child's deafness work for you?

In successful families, the behaviors stemming from the unpleasant feelings present in the initial stages of the grief process are reframed and transformed into positive action. The transformation occurs as the family gains confidence and as the professional listens sensitively in a positive, affirming manner. Thus, the anger is transformed into an energy that can work for the child, the guilt becomes commitment, the feelings of inadequacy and confusion become the impetus to learn, and the feeling of vulnerability initiates a restructuring of priorities.

The Group

There is probably no greater gift that a professional can give to families than to provide them with a support group. Groups are marvelous vehicles for learning and emotional support as one goes through the grief process. Most support groups in our field are composed of parents, although there are grandparents' groups and siblings' groups as well. The benefits for everyone are the same. In a well-managed group, which is not content dominated, group members can recognize the universality of their feelings; they can come to appreciate that other people in a similar position have similar feelings. Very often, family members feel that something is wrong with them because they have such powerful emotions that do not conform to conventional expectations; e.g., anger and fear, in particular. It is with relief that they realize that other people feel the same way. Within the context of a group, they can learn something no professional can teach them—that they are not alone

The group also gives the participants the opportunity to help one another. As has been discussed, family members so often are the recipients of direct help from others that their self-esteem is diminished; within a group of peers, they have as much opportunity to help as to be helped, and this tends to enhance self-esteem.

The group also becomes a powerful vehicle for imparting information. Working with groups, I am always astonished at how much individuals already know, and I seldom leave a group without having learned something. The collective wisdom within a group is greater than the knowledge of any one participant.

The support group needs to be a fundamental part of any habilitation program for families. The Wagners, the Murphys, and the Marshalls felt strongly that the parent group was very important to them. Invariably, it is the element of the Emerson program that parents remember.

There is much more to the group process than can be covered within the scope of a chapter. Interested readers can pursue this fascinating subject area further by examining Luterman (1984) or, better yet, by reading Yalom (1975).

The Successful Professional

All that has been said about the feelings and treatment of family members applies equally to the professionals. The feelings the parents experience also are a part of the professional's reaction; under the affect skin, we are all brothers and sisters. Audiologists often feel overwhelmed by the responsibility of determining the hearing status of a young child and guiding the parents to a satisfactory solution. All professionals feel anger. They feel anger at parents for not following through on a recommended course of action. They feel rage, frustration, and sometimes despair when they cannot make things better for the child or family or when they can't locate an appropriate placement. They feel an anger toward other professionals who treat the families insensitively or inappropriately.

Guilt also is part of the professional's experience; I know of no responsible, competent professionals who have no regrets about some families with whom they have worked. Mistakes are an inevitable part of all growing professionals. In one sense, mistakes are ''nuggets of gold,'' they are markers for what needs to be learned, they indicate the direction in which growth is needed. I have learned far more from my mistakes than I have from my successes. My success I take for granted; my mistakes spur me on to new learning. Mistakes are seldom seen as valuable by professionals. I think this emanates from an educational system that penalizes mistakes very heavily. Consequently, professionals are often needlessly burdened by guilt for their errors, which limits severely their willingness to take risks and to grow professionally.

All professionals who work with disabled people become acutely aware of their own vulnerability. One cannot help but do this when one sees, day in and day out, handicapped individuals. Awareness of one's vulnerability can lead to very positive behavior. When we recognize our vulnerability, we can begin to reorder our priorities. We don't waste time and we recognize and appreciate what is truly important.

Always at issue for me is the personal growth of the professional. The personal being of the professional is by far the most important clinical tool in amelioration of the child's deafness and in helping the family cope with the deafness. Professionals need to pay attention to their own personal growth and personal congruence because, as they feel secure and loving towards themselves, they can accept and love others. When professionals are internally structured, they can allow others to have freedom.

As a profession, we need to pay attention to our need to be needed, which leads to behaviors that interfere with good helping. Professionals with an unchecked need to be needed are loathe to give up the child or the credit for helping the child. Secure professionals can allow the parents to be smart and can diminish their obvious importance to the families. As a profession, we need to be concerned about promoting the personal growth of all audiologists and teachers. We need to examine clinical training procedures that tend to look at deficits and penalize mistakes. We need to select students in training programs with an eye towards helping them develop their interpersonal skills and their personal congruence. Lastly, we need to incorporate opportunities for personal growth within training programs.

Frequently, when the feelings and experiences surrounding

deafness in children are discussed, the painful and negative emotions are emphasized; seldom are the positive feelings and experiences described. To be sure, a great deal of pain and stress must be endured in coming to grips with having a hearing-impaired child, but what is often overlooked is the marvelous opportunities for joy and growth that also are present. I frequently tell parents that this child comes bearing a gift that is buried under a great deal of pain and stress. It is their lifelong job to find that gift. Many parents come through the experience of having a deaf child with a clearer sense of themselves and their own worth. They develop a clearer sense of their priorities than they had before their child was diagnosed as hearing impaired. Many parents find that their child's deafness gives their lives meaning and direction. Their joy stems from actively participating in their child's growth. They take nothing for granted. They can see what needs to be done and they can rejoice when a milestone is reached. They also know that they had a direct hand in reaching that milestone. As Bertrand Russell said, "To be without some of the things you want is an indispensable part of happiness."

There also is joy and satisfaction for the professional who knows that a good job has been done in helping the families grow and cope with their children's handicaps. My most meaningful clinical experiences have been in the intimate relationships that I have had with parents of hearing-impaired children; it is very gratifying to witness and participate actively in people's growing and reaching their potential. I willingly will share some of their pain if they will share some of their joy with me. Over the years, I number among my best friends members of several families with whom I have worked. You, the reader, have met some of them within these pages.

One mother summarized the positive aspects of her experience:

It made you more aware of things. More appreciative. . . . It made me kind of stop and smell the flowers a lot more than I would before. I was always kind of rushing around and hurrying and not stopping . . . stopping as much as I do now. I'm just kind of enjoying everything as much as possible because you just realize, I don't know, maybe your vulnerability. Who knows what's going to happen next, so you might as well enjoy now. I used to think that that could never happen to me . . . but I don't feel that way anymore. Not in a real negative, pessimistic kind of thing, but it's life and you have no control over it, so you might as well appreciate what you have. Make the best of it.

REFERENCES

Chinn, P., Winn, S., & Walters, R. (1978). *Two-way talking with parents of special children*. St. Louis: C. V. Mosby Co.

Featherstone, H. (1980). *A difference in the family*. New York: Basic Books.

Gallagher, S. S., Cross, A., & Scharfman, W. (1981). Parental adaptation to a young handicapped child: The father's role. *Journal of the Division of Early Childhood, 3*, 3–14.

Harvey, M. (1984). Family therapy with deaf persons: The systematic utilization of an interpreter. *Family Process, 23*, 205–213.

Lavell, N. & Keogh, B. (1980). Expectation and attribution of parents of handicapped children. In S. S. Gallagher (Ed.), *Parents and families of handicapped children*. San Francisco: Josey-Bass, Inc.

LeMaistre, J. (1985). *Beyond rage*. Oak Park, IL: Alpine Guild.

Longo, D. & Bond, L. (1984). Families of the handicapped child: Research and practice. *Family Relations, 33*, 57–65.

Luterman, D. (1984). *Counseling the communicatively disordered and their families*. Boston: Little, Brown, Inc.

Mendelsohn, M., & Rozek, F. (1983). Denying disability: The case of deafness. *Family Systems Medicine, 1*, 37–47.

Minuchin, S., Rosman, B., & Baker, L. (1978). *Psychosomatic families*. Cambridge, MA: Harvard University Press.

Robinson, L., & Weathers, O. (1974). Psychotherapeutic intervention. *American Annals of the Deaf, 119*, 325–330.

Sandow, S., & Clarke D. B. (1977). Home intervention with parents of severely subnormal, pre-school children: An interim report. *Child Care, Health and Development, 4*, 29–39.

Shapiro, R. S., & Harris, R. (1976). Family therapy in treatment of the deaf. *Family Process, 15*, 83–97.

Venters, M. (1981). Familial coping with chronic and severe childhood illness: The case of cystic fibrosis. *Social Science and Medicine, 15A*, 289–297.

Williams, D. M., & Darbyshire, J. (1982). Diagnosis of deafness: A study of family responses and needs. *Volta Review, 84*, 24–30.

Yalom, I. (1975). *The theory and practice of group psychotherapy*. New York: Basic Books.

INDEX

A

Adaptation to crisis of having handicapped child, major styles of, 50–51

Affectional needs
of deaf child, 37–38
of hearing child, 33–34

Affiliation
of the deaf child, 35–37
dealing with in Murphy family, 69
of the hearing child, 32–33

Anger
as grandparent's reaction to deaf child, 96
as parental reaction to child's deafness, 42
as sibling response to deaf child, 78

Anorexia, 3

Anxiety, as parental reaction to child's deafness, 41

B

Beck Depression Inventory, 76

Boundaries of family
deaf child's interference of, 101–102
extrafamilial, 99–100
in sibling subsystem, 102

C

Cerebral palsy, 44, 75
severe, 105

Change
from extrafamilial sources, 100
in the family, 100–101

Child Care Index, 76

Child
deaf
affectional needs of, 37–38
affiliation of, 35–37

119

Date Due